Every year throughout the world, an estimated three-quarters of a million people take their own life, and in many countries this is the leading cause of death in the 25–34 age group. Suicide and attempted suicide therefore at some time affect the lives of a significant proportion of the population and are problems of major concern for health-care professionals, as well as for the family and friends of the suicide victim. However, suicide continues to carry the stigma of shame, creating barriers to the promotion of knowledge and understanding about why people attempt suicide and how it can be prevented.

Professor Nils Retterstøl is a world expert in this field, and in this book, translated and expanded from his original Norwegian text, he presents the issues related to the growing problem of suicide and suicidal attempts. The book considers the range of factors which underlie the problem, including social and cultural circumstances, psychological factors, psychiatric disorders and somatic conditions. Methods of evaluating the suicide risk are discussed and approaches to treatment and prevention are presented, with regard to both psychotherapeutic methods and the newer pharmacological and biological practices. Professor Retterstøl also presents a graphic account of the consequences of suicide for the survivor, exemplified by his own experiences of follow-up. Later chapters are concerned with the problems faced by the relatives of people who have committed suicide and the support which they require; the final chapter considers suicide prevention measures on an individual, local, national and international basis.

Placing the subject in an international context, Professor Retterstøl provides a sensitive and enlightening account of the problem of suicide and attempted suicide in today's societies. This pioneering book is a unique source of information which will be of the greatest value to all clinicians, health-care professionals and lay-people, working with suicidal patients and their families.

Suicide

Suicide

A European Perspective

NILS RETTERSTØL

Gaustad Hospital, University of Oslo, Oslo, Norway

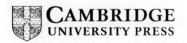

CAMBRIDGE
UNIVERSITY PRESS

Published by the Press Syndicate of the University of Cambridge
The Pitt Building, Trumpington Street, Cambridge CB2 1RP
40 West 20th Street, New York, NY 10011-4211, USA
10 Stamford Road, Oakleigh, Melbourne 3166, Australia

First published in Norwegian as *Selvmord* by Universitetsforlaget, Oslo
1970, fourth edition 1990, and © Universitetsforlaget 1970, 1978, 1985, 1990

First published in English by Cambridge University Press 1993 as *Suicide: a European perspective*
English translation © Cambridge University Press 1993

Printed in Great Britain at the University Press, Cambridge

A catalogue record for this book is available from the British Library

Library of Congress cataloguing in publication data

Retterstøl, Nils, 1924–
    Suicide : a European perspective / Nils Retterstøl.
        p.   cm.
    Includes bibliographical references and index.
    ISBN 0-521-42099-7
    1. Suicide.   I. Title.
HV 6545.R415   1993
362.2'8'094–dc20   92-39458   CIP

ISBN 0 521 42099 7 hardback

Contents

Preface

This book was originally written in Norwegian, and was widely read in the Scandinavian countries. The first edition was published in 1970. New, heavily revised editions then appeared in 1978, 1985 and 1990. Over the intervening period, rapid developments have taken place in suicidology, the science of self-destructive behaviour. It seems clear that suicide is becoming more prevalent, not just in Norway but throughout Europe and in the rest of the world.

Around the world, some 2000 people end their lives through suicide every day, representing a toll of 80–100 deaths per hour. In many countries, suicide is the leading cause of death in the 25–34 age group. In all, around three-quarters of a million people die at their own hands every year. In Europe it is estimated, by the World Health Organization, that 135,000 people per year take their own life. This is only part of the suicide problem.

Around 10 to 15 times as many people make non-fatal suicidal attempts – or perform parasuicidal acts. In the young, the ratio may be 20–40 attempts to one suicide and in the elderly this can be 3:1. This means that every year, 10 to 20 million people deliberately harm themselves in this way. In addition, there will be partners, children and friends who suffer because of a person committing or attempting suicide. If it is assumed there are five people around each deceased person, some four million people annually will be confronted with the emotional consequences of losing someone through the suicidal act. It may take years to complete the mourning process. Some 50 to 100 million people around those who attempt suicide will be affected.

In addition to suicide and suicide attempts, many, and perhaps most, of us have had suicidal thoughts on one or more occasions in our lives. Many threaten to take their own lives. It is said that many marriages have been made under the threat of suicide from one of the partners, and many marriages are kept going by such threats.

Suicide is a central human problem, in practice one of importance to most people. Strong taboos continue to exist on suicidal matters. These taboos have to be broken down. One of the aims of this book is to shed light on suicide and suicidal problems – for both professionals and laypeople.

The taboos have to be broken down if we are to be able to give better treatment and show greater understanding to the suicidal person, and if we are to reduce the alarming number of suicides.

A great deal of new material has appeared on the causal factors of suicide and attempted suicide. New guidelines have been issued for treatment and prevention, guidelines which are presented in this book. New material has also appeared on educational activity in relation to the suicide problem and the significance of this, as well as on the unfortunate consequences of more sensationalist coverage of suicide in the mass media.

As a clinical psychiatrist for almost 40 years, I have seen the key role that the suicide problem plays in psychiatric work. Assessing the danger of suicide is one of the most difficult and challenging tasks a doctor, and particularly a clinical psychiatrist, has to face. All psychiatrists will encounter incorrect assessments in this area during their lifetimes, with the tragic consequences this can have for the individual and his or her nearest and dearest. The same type of problem faces clinical psychologists, social workers, nurses and other interdisciplinary members of staff every day. It is necessary to expand knowledge of suicidology among all who work in the health-care professions, since the assessment depends not just on intuition and clinical insight but also to a great extent on knowledge.

My aim in writing this book is to help raise the level of knowledge on the subject of suicidology in the health-care professions and the general public. I also wish to pass on opinions from international psychiatry. In June 1989 I was elected President of the International Association for Suicide Prevention and Crisis Intervention in Brussels. I have been on the Board of this organization for a number of years, and have also had the privilege of working with key specialists throughout the world. There can be little doubt that one of the most important preventive measures that can be taken today is to increase knowledge on the subject of suicidology and pass this knowledge on to health-care practitioners and the general public. I hope that this book will offer useful information and valuable findings to doctors, psychologists, nurses, clergy, social workers and the many interdisciplinary members of staff whose work involves dealing with people at risk of suicide. I hope that I have succeeded in keeping the book at a sufficiently simple linguistic level for it to be read with benefit by non-specialists as well as specialists.

The Cambridge University Press felt that this book would be of interest to a wider readership than a Scandinavian language could give it. The 1990 edition of the book has therefore been updated and translated into English. A few local Norwegian problems have been taken out, European data added, and some material of greater relevance to the British and American situation has been incorporated. It is my hope that useful material can also be passed on to an international public.

The use of 'he' has been adopted throughout this book, where necessary, as to use the term he/she each time becomes rather clumsy, so I apologise now for any offence that may be caused to readers.

I wish to thank Randi Remen of Gaustad Hospital, Oslo, for excellent secretarial help in the preparation of the manuscript, Finn Gjertsen of the Norwegian Central Bureau of Statistics, Oslo, for help with the statistical work, Dr Richard Barling of the Cambridge University Press for efficient work in editing the English edition, Robert Williams MA, MIL, MITI for conscientious work on the translation from Norwegian to English and Rita Owen for her many suggested improvements to the manuscript.

Nils Retterstøl, Oslo, 1992

1

Introduction – definitions

Suicide is probably the most personal act anyone can perform. Few acts have such deep roots in social and human conditions, or have such far reaching consequences. No other act has such great consequences for oneself. Suicide affects the single individual who takes his life, it affects this person's immediate circle and it affects the local community as well as the wider community. It is of interest to people of very different categories: doctors, psychologists, social workers, nurses, sociologists, lawyers, clergymen, teachers, the police, writers, philosophers and politicians, but it is also of interest to all ordinary members of the public. Many of us have known people who have committed suicide or who have attempted to do so. It may be anticipated that everyone at intolerable and difficult moments in his or her life will entertain the idea that it might be best to put an end to it all. Suicidal thoughts, threats and attempted suicide are common general human phenomena. I do not know of any culture in which suicide does not occur. Suicide is a human phenomenon; it is not known among other animals.

In Norway around 650 people are known to die annually through suicide (in 1991 the figure was 675). This is what the official death statistics from the Central Bureau of Statistics tell us. There are many suicides which are not recorded but where the cause of death is listed as something else. This may be partly due to there being doubt as to whether the person in question himself wanted to take his life, whether it was chance circumstances that caused the death, or whether it was simply an accident. The doctor who issues the death certificate will tend to give the 'benefit' of the doubt to the deceased by indicating a different diagnosis. Causes of death such as poisoning or drowning may be listed in cases

1

where the poisoning or drowning was self-inflicted, but where there is no definite proof of this. However, we must also be aware that suicide may occasionally be recorded where the death perhaps deep down was not actually intended. It is a commonly held view on the basis of international surveys that the 'correct' number of suicides in a population is 25% higher than that officially registered. This would suggest that there are at present 900 cases of suicide per year in Norway, which means there are more than two suicides per day.

Some definitions of terms to which I shall frequently return in this book, terms which are central to the study of suicide are presented below.

Suicide

A common definition is as follows:

- An act with a fatal outcome,
  that is deliberately initiated and performed by the deceased him- or herself,
  in the knowledge or expectation of its fatal outcome,
  the outcome being considered by the actor as instrumental in bringing about desired changes in consciousness and/or social conditions

definition

A further definition:

- Suicide is a self-inflicted, life-threatening act which results in death.

A third is the proposal the World Health Organization (WHO) has made for a new definition of suicide:

- Suicide is an act with a fatal outcome which the deceased, with the knowledge and expectation of a fatal outcome, had himself planned and carried out with the object of bringing about the changes desired by the deceased.

An attempt at a definition is made by a Norwegian team of sociologists (Hammerlin & Enerstvedt, 1988):

- Suicide is an activity which involves acts with the aim and result of one's own biological death on the basis of social, specific historical motives.

Attempted suicide

The following definitions have been proposed on the basis of considerations corresponding to those underlying the definitions of suicide:

- By attempted suicide we understand a conscious and voluntary act which the individual has undertaken in order to injure himself, and which the individual could not have been entirely certain of surviving, but where the injury has not led to death.
- A self-inflicted, life-threatening act which does not result in death.
- An acute, consciously self-destructive act which does not lead to death.
- Attempted suicide comprises situations in which a person has displayed actual or apparent life-threatening behaviour with the purpose of putting his or her life at risk or of giving the appearance of such a purpose, but which has not resulted in death.
- Attempted suicide is an activity which involves acts of intentional self-injury and with the object of death, but where the result is not death (Hammerlin & Enersvedt, 1988).

Some use the word parasuicide instead of the term *attempted suicide* to express the fact that it is a phenomenon which is close to or similar to suicide but nevertheless different.

The following proposed definition of attempted suicide is put forward in the WHO (WHO, 1986) proposals for a new classification list:

- A non-habitual act with non-fatal outcome,
  that is deliberately initiated and performed by the individual involved,
  that causes self-harm, or without intervention from others will do so, or consists of ingesting a substance in excess of its generally recognised therapeutic dosage.

Parasuicide is defined as follows:

- A non-habitual act with non-fatal outcome,
  that is deliberately initiated and performed by the individual involved *in expectation of such an outcome*,
  that causes self-harm, or without intervention from others will do so, or consists of ingesting a substance in excess of its generally recognised therapeutic dosage,
  the outcome being considered by the actor as instrumental in bringing about desired changes in expectancies and/or social condition.

Comment

The consciously self-destructive purpose in both suicide and attempted suicide may be vague and accompanied by doubt or ambivalence. It is often chance factors that decide whether the outcome is fatal or whether the person in question survives. Follow-up studies show that by far the majority of those who survive a suicidal attempt do not make any further attempts at suicide.

Suicidal thoughts

These comprise behaviour that can be directly observed where the person concerned states that he or she is thinking about putting an end to his or her life. The category of suicidal thoughts includes thoughts which are spontaneously reported to others, or which are confirmed when the person concerned is asked.

Suicidal messages

These are signs of a tendency towards suicide which are communicated to the world at large through speech, behaviour or action. These messages may be conscious or unconscious for the person issuing them.

Suicidal threats

These are threats that an individual wants to take his or her own life, usually if wishes are not respected or conditions are not met.

Suicidal risk

This is the judgment made by another person, often a specialist, who attempts to assess the likelihood of the person concerned taking his or her own life on the basis of a knowledge of the background, life situation, pathological features of the person, statistical data and the reactions of those around the person.

Suicidal process

This is a term which describes suicidal behaviour as a development from suicidal thoughts and attempted suicide through to accomplished suicide. During the course of this process the suicidal tendency may be greater or lesser and develop in a positive or negative direction. Whether people take the ultimate step and take their own lives, or attempt to do so, issue threats or harbour suicidal thoughts, they are all humans in distress and difficulty. The suicidal acts or patterns of behaviour which are associated with suicide are usually preceded by a long period of development which often has its origins back in childhood. The self-destructive act has come as a reaction to a situation which has involved isolation, humiliation, loss of self-esteem, loss of love and affection, provocation of insecurity, etc. The external situation has often been 'the straw which has broken the camel's already straining back'.   .

Suicide rate

This term is used to refer to the number of suicides registered per 100,000 people in a population over the course of one year. The registered cases of suicide will be those where the doctor has given suicide as the cause of death, and where the death certificate has given a central registration office reason to believe that suicide has been the cause of death. As already mentioned, the registered number of suicides is probably considerably lower than the true number – an underestimate of 25% is usually anticipated.

Rate of attempted suicide

The problem of suicide is on a completely different scale than the suicide figures suggest. It is estimated that around ten times as many people unsuccessfully attempt suicide. In Norway there is no central registration of the rate of attempted suicides and is therefore best analysed through the rate of attempted suicide in a limited area, for example within a particular sector of a population. However, only the number of cases which have resulted in hospital admissions or out-patient treatment in hospitals will generally be recorded. It is thought that a considerable number of people who attempt suicide are never treated in any medical institution.

The 'chronically suicidal'

These are a group of people who over a long period take their own lives through their life-style: daredevils who repeatedly take risks and survive one accident after another (*accident proneness*), alcohol and drug abusers who in the long run shorten their lives by several years, and also people who neglect to have themselves treated for their physical disorders. The category of the *chronically suicidal* also includes those people who resolve their conflicts by attempting suicide, people who make repeated attempts at suicide and are admitted to hospital wards, and in some cases try the patience of those who treat them.

Once-off phenomenon – pattern of behaviour

Suicidal acts may be a *once-off* phenomenon in a particularly deadlocked and difficult life situation. They can also be patterns of behaviour which follow the individual in difficult phases of his or her life. Attempted suicide in people of this type can represent an escape from the problems they cannot overcome by more rational or adequate methods.

Means of communication – means of aggression

For many people, attempted suicide represents a means of communication with the world at large. Suicidal behaviour is used to signal to an individual's immediate circle that he is in distress and needs help. For others, attempted suicide may be a *means of aggression*, a way of punishing their immediate circle. It has been said that whilst marital problems in the past used to be resolved with the aid of china – by throwing cups at the wall – the same is done today with the aid of the medicine cabinet.

Double suicide

This is when two people both of whom are set on committing suicide together. Such cases are more common in poetry and prose than in reality.

Extended suicide

Also known as complex suicide, is said to take place when one or more persons against their will are involved in the death. It is usually marriage partners or children who are affected, and family tragedies of this kind can develop in connection with mental illness. The patient's thoughts are based on dreadful impending catastrophes, which he wishes to prevent himself and his nearest and dearest from experiencing.

Euthanasia

Active euthanasia, also known as mercy killing, is a form of suicidal act. The death-bringing act is carried out by someone else on the wishes of a person who is suffering from a fatal or assumed fatal illness, to save the patient from a painful death or a protracted fight against death. This problem is discussed later in the book.

Victim-precipitated homicide

The expression is used in relation to homicides where the victim himself is the one who directly and positively induced the criminal act. The victim has usually been the first to use physical form and provoked the murder by directly challenging his opponent to use violence (e.g. threatening him with a knife or pistol).

Finally some special forms of suicide described by the American psychiatrist Karl Menninger (1938) must be mentioned.

Focal (local) suicide

This refers to certain forms of self-destruction such as where mental patients destroy parts of their bodies or people keep subjecting themselves to new operations to have organs removed because of symptoms they believe come from these organs. In the USA there are a number of people who have several organs removed over an extended period because of symptoms which in the long-term perspective will be assumed to be due to neurosis. Menninger mentions as the most innocent forms of local suicide such general phenomena as nail-biting, finger-biting, scratching and hair-plucking. He also categorises impotence, including frigidity, in this way. This is because he looks at these phenomena as a form of self-induced inhibition localised in the genital organs. It is a form of functional destruction of these parts of the body.

Organic suicide

Finally, Menninger talks of 'organic suicide', represented by organic diseases that he believes, in a good many cases, may be due to unconscious conflicts which are linked to aggressive, self-punishing and self-destructive tendencies. People may also neglect to have themselves treated for a physical disorder, for example, not taking insulin in diabetes.

I have mentioned Menninger's hypotheses not because they are generally accepted or scientifically verified but because they offer new, interesting and rewarding perspectives on the problem of suicide, which is thus considered in an even wider perspective than that traditionally adopted.

Chronic suicide

The direct self-destructive act here takes place over a long period. Suicide is committed, as it were, inch by inch. Ascetism and martyrdom are placed under this heading, as are alcohol and drug abuse and antisocial behaviour.

Many factors – suicidal acts as acts with multifactorial causes

It is rare to be able to point to a single factor which alone has brought about a suicide or an attempted suicide. A number of factors that have conspired will generally be found. These may be predisposing factors which have developed for example during a difficult and deadlocked childhood, triggering factors in the practical life situation or a mental disorder which has developed as a consequence of these, and which has sucked the individual into a vicious circle. Nor can there generally be said to be a problem of pure aggression or a pure appeal function, both parts being present in varying proportions.

2

Suicide from the perspective of cultural history

Many books have been written about suicide from the perspective of cultural history. If viewed from the standpoint of cultural history, a distinction can quickly be made between two forms of suicide: social or institutionalised suicide, and individual or personal suicide.

Social or institutionalised suicide

This is a form of self-destruction which society almost demands as a consequence of the identification of the individual with his group. Throughout history this type of suicide can be recognised in many cultures. Examples of such types of suicide are the death of the widow, servant or slave in connection with that of the husband or master. Other examples can be taken from countries where famine and death have prevailed, and where the old or sick were expected to sacrifice themselves so that the younger and healthier should survive. When the elderly could no longer follow the tribe, they would be left behind, either on their own initiative or that of the tribe. In some cultures suicide has been expected in humiliating situations or defeat, such as from a general who has lost an important battle.

Personal or individual suicide

This has often emerged from the same causal mechanisms as we see today in suicide – a deadlocked or difficult life situation which an individual is unable to resolve by normal methods, escape mechanisms, aggression, or mental illness.

I shall first look at suicide in non-western cultural communities and then discuss suicide within the Judaeo-Christian cultural community.

Hinduism

Eastern religions, and particularly Hinduism, have not had the traditionally negative view of suicide which are held in the West. In the old books of the Veda, suicide was permitted for religious reasons. The best sacrifice that could be made was one's own life. On the other hand, there was also strong opposition in the Upanishads (the Holy Scriptures) to suicide, which was condemned. In one of the Upanishads it is stated that 'he who takes his own life will enter the sunless areas covered by impenetrable darkness after death'. In Hinduism *suttee* or *sati* (widow-burning) was recognised, institutionalised and sanctioned until modern times.

Although the oldest scripture of the Brahmins, the Rig-Veda, does not contain any rules on suttee, it has been a common tradition in the Hindu religion that voluntary death represented a definite route to salvation for the widow. According to the Hindu religion it is the self – we could almost say the soul – which survives whilst the body perishes. A verse in one of the Upanishads states that 'it is the body that dies when it is left by the self, the self does not die'. By joining her husband on the funeral-pyre, the widow could atone for the husband's sins, free him of punishment and clear the way to a better life both for him and for herself. The widow had to undergo a number of rituals beforehand. After her husband died she had a day in which to decide whether she wanted to commit suttee. Once she had expressed her decision to do so, she could not withdraw with her honour intact. The act was highly respected by fellow citizens. The tradition was prohibited in India and declared a crime in 1892. Sporadic cases of widow-burning have nevertheless occurred right up to the present, particularly in country districts.

Suicide by starvation has also been sanctioned by religious groups in Indian culture. This form of suicide was known as *sallekhana* and was often performed by ascetics. Famine as a political weapon was developed on this basis by Mahatma Gandhi in his spiritual fight against British rule in India. In more recent times this type of fasting has ended in death in several cases, sometimes in the struggles of minority groups, or in the fight against what has been felt to be political injustice. Threats of fasting to death are believed still to be common in India today.

Buddhism

In the Buddhist religion too, suicide was regarded as correct in certain circumstances, and consistent with the objective of human life according to this religion: needs, ambitions and strong feelings should be extinguished. The best self-sacrifice may be to free oneself of one's own existence. It may be better to give one's body than to give alms. It is more worthy to burn one's own body that to light lamps on a shrine.

In China special motives for suicide were particularly recognised – the general who killed himself after a lost battle, the deposed statesman who protested against official policy by committing suicide, people who committed suicide in memory of their deceased father or another ancestor. If one had lost face through an infringement of the law or a loss, suicide was an accepted solution. If the criminal was a person of high rank, it was not uncommon for the Emperor to send him a yellow silk scarf to hang himself with, so that he could in this way avoid criminal prosecution, disgrace and possibly a death sentence. Many a Chinese general has had a yellow silk scarf sent to him by the Emperor. Suicide as an act of revenge against someone who has committed an injustice against one is also well known from China. Responsibility for the deed was then transferred to the other person, and one's soul could pursue the enemy better than one could as a living person.

However, the Buddhist attitude towards suicide is generally negative. According to Buddhist teaching, human life is primarily one of suffering and stress, and it is one of man's duties to withstand this suffering. It will be difficult for someone who takes his life to free himself of such suffering to be reincarnated. Under Confucian doctrine, one must not destroy one's body, not even the hair or skin, because it is given to one by one's ancestors. With the strict family obligations one has under this doctrine, self-destructive behaviour is unacceptable. Suicide is prohibited according to the teachings of Confucius, except in cases where one has to show one's loyalty to an organisation to which one belongs.

Japanese culture

Suicide has been more involved in national tradition in Japan than elsewhere. Japanese religion is based partly on Shintoism and partly on Buddhism. The traditional rituals of *seppuku* and *hara-kiri* gradually developed. It was in the higher social classes, chiefly the nobility and the military (the Samurai) that these forms of suicide were practised.

Hara-kiri originated a thousand years ago, in the early stages of feudalism in Japan. It was originally an honourable form of suicide to avoid being captured. The person concerned first thrust a short sword into the left side of his abdomen, moved it across to the right and pulled it out. He then thrust it into his midriff and cut vertically upwards. Finally he slit his throat. This act was seen as a form of bravery. One could also be condemned to commit hara-kiri. Suicide could thus be either compulsory or voluntary. Compulsory suicide was ordered for nobles, who could atone for their criminal acts or loss of face with their swords. Voluntary hara-kiri tended to be carried out as a protest against a superior or ruler, or in sorrow over the death of this person. Although both forms of hara-kiri were forbidden by law in 1868, they are still practised. Hara-kiri is performed according to a fixed ceremony, with a particular type of knife, and usually with an assistant present. The author has himself seen patients admitted for emergency treatment at the Nippon Medical School in Tokyo after they have unsuccessfully attempted to commit hara-kiri.

Suicide performed after the death of one's superior is known as *junshi*. Junshi was practised after a person of high status died, and the person who committed junshi believed that the spirit of the superior concerned would be necessary for him in life after death. A modern example of junshi was that of General Nogi and his wife, who practised this form of suicide after the death of the Emperor Meiji in 1912.

It is well known that Japanese culture has been favourable towards suicide. During the Second World War the Japanese had no difficulty in recruiting suicide servicemen for one-man aircraft, the kamikaze pilots, who crashed themselves and their machines, packed with explosive, into enemy targets. There were also one-man submarines, kaiten.

Japan has traditionally been very high in world suicide statistics. Since the Second World War, Japan has been exposed to a considerable degree of Americanisation and western influence. An increase in the suicide rate had been expected, as commonly occurs when two cultures collide. In Japan the opposite was found. Although the suicide rate did rise slightly in the first five years after the end of the Second World War, it then fell, so that the Japanese suicide rate today is at the middle level internationally. One aspect is, however, characteristic: the ratio between men and women in Japan is 1:1, whilst the ratio in most western countries is 3:1 or 2:1, with a clear preponderance of male suicides. Suicide is the most common cause of death among young Japanese women. In most western countries there is a clear clustering of suicides in cities and built-up areas but this is not the case in Japan. There has, however, been an increase in the suicide rate in Japan as there has been in Europe.

Islam

No religion has had a more condemnatory attitude towards suicide than Islam. Mohammed declared that God had allotted to each human being its dignity, Kismet, and that He alone determined the time when the person would die. One of the main doctrines of Islam is that God's will is expressed in various ways, and that man has to subjugate oneself to His will at all times. One disregards God's will if one commits suicide. Suicide is therefore considered a very serious crime in Islam, worse than murder.

'Primitive cultures' – collisions of cultures

It has been claimed that suicide does not occur in more 'primitive' cultures. This is, however, incorrect. As far as is known, there is no culture that is free of suicide.

In some cultures suicide is a way of expressing anger or vengeance, based on personal motives. The form in which it is expressed may be precisely described through regulations and customs. In primitive cultures the motives have often been the desire to preserve honour and dignity or prove that one was not a coward. It was also accepted that suicide could be committed because of severe pain or helplessness in old age or infirmity. In many cultures it has also been viewed as a reasonable act by a woman if her virtue was in danger, if she had been subjected to rape, or for a man if he wanted to avoid personal humiliation by falling into the hands of the enemy. It could also be an expression of an unwillingness to bear the burden of being separated from a loved one in extreme circumstances or death. Feelings of shame and vengeance are common motives for suicide in 'primitive' cultures. The revenge which follows from 'killing oneself over the head of another' is often thought of as being exacted by the spirit of the dead person. It is not unusual in 'primitive' societies for old members of a tribe to take their own lives so that they do not carry on living as weak and miserable beings who are a burden on the community. These motives are said to occur among the Eskimos.

The suicide rate, however, usually rises when the 'primitive' culture meets our so-called civilisation. A clash of this kind often leads to a disintegration of old social norms, the abuse of alcohol and drugs, the break-up of families and promiscuity. One example which is often quoted these days is that of Greenland, which now appears to have the highest suicide rate in the world, in 1987 it was recorded as 127 per 100,000 people per year (Ministry of Health, 1987). The suicide rate is also extremely high among Native Americans on reservations in the USA. Their life-style has to be re-arranged when they are placed on reservations, and many of their ancient traditions become meaningless. At the same time, the inhabitants lack the stimulus of belonging to the society which surrounds them and adopting its norms.

The Graeco-Roman cultural community

Ancient Greece

In Ancient Greece suicide was regarded as a shameful act. A person who had committed suicide was not granted the death ritual which was customary for ordinary citizens. Life was a gift which was given by the gods, and life and death were subjugated to the will of the gods. Suicide was seen as a form of rebellion against the gods. Since people were the property of the gods, suicide would therefore cause harm to the gods.

Plato says in one of his writings that a person who has committed suicide should be buried without any marks of respect at a lonely place where no monument can be erected on the place of burial. In his time the bodies of those who had committed suicide were usually burnt outside the towns, and the hand was cut off and buried separately. Aristotle also denounced suicide. He stated emphatically that it was also a sin of weakness against the fatherland – since man owes his life to his father-land, an act by which one voluntarily renounces this life is in reality a criminal dereliction of one's clear civic duties. Authors such as Plutarch, Euripides and Virgil denounced suicide as a cowardly and wretched act, unworthy of man.

There were nevertheless examples of suicide which were regarded as an heroic act in Ancient Greece: Kodios, who sacrificed his life to save Athens from the Lacedaemonians, and Themistocles who preferred to poison himself rather than lead the Persians against his compatriots.

The Stoic School

Was founded in Greece by Zenon around 400 BC and flourished in the Roman Empire. There were distinct views on suicide in the Stoic School. In some situations suicide was defended as an act worthy of respect:

(1) When a service is done for others by committing suicide, e.g. for the fatherland.
(2) When the perpetrator, by committing suicide, avoids being forced to perform an unlawful or morally reprehensible act.
(3) When poverty, chronic disease or mental illness makes death more attractive than life.

The highest law of the Stoics was to live in accordance with nature and reason. Pliny the Elder considered the existence of poisonous herbs to be royal and divine proof that man could allow himself to die without pain. The Stoic Seneca argued for suicide as a method of escape or to put an end to suffering, particularly the weakness of old age and physical decline.

Zenon, the founder of Stoic philosophy, had found life worth living right up to the age of 98. He then fell and dislocated a big toe. This unsettled him to such an extent that he no longer found life worth living, and went home and hanged himself. Seneca, who had been the tutor of the Emperor Nero, and who was a leading representative of the Stoic school, took his own life when he fell into disgrace with the tyrant. He was followed into death by his wife.

Both Pliny the Elder and his nephew Pliny the Younger had a stoical attitude towards suicide. They believed that it was right to weigh up the motives for and against when life became difficult and illnesses many. A plus and minus account was drawn up. 'Voluntarily weighing up the motives for and against, and then on the basis of the advice deciding on life or death, is the decision of a great soul.'

An example of a cool and considered suicidal act which merited honour and was an expression of patriotism was the death of Cato of Utica. He stabbed himself to death rather than live under the tyrannical rule of Caesar, prompted by concern for his fatherland and by his firm principles. Caesar was so impressed with this act that he made the following pronouncement: 'Cato, I envy you your death in the same way that you have envied me my power to preserve your life'.

The Stoics were also pre-occupied with the way in which suicide was to be carried out – it should preferably be done quietly, without theatrical gestures.

The Cynical and Epicurean schools. Roman legislation

The Cynical and Epicurean schools of philosophy accepted suicide under certain circumstances. As the laws on suicide gradually took shape in the ancient Roman Empire, economic considerations came into the picture, for example, the suicide of a slave meant a significant economic burden for the master, and the suicide of a soldier weakened the Roman armies. Attempted suicide was a punishable offence. For a soldier the penalty could be death, because attempted suicide was equated with desertion. The property of a person who had committed suicide was confiscated – slaves were considered as property and were, therefore not allowed to commit suicide. However, a heroic sacrificial suicide for the State was highly regarded. In the ancient Roman Empire there was a positive attitude towards suicide which was carried out in order to avoid disgrace, avoid pain, express sorrow over the loss of a loved one, or was performed in order to serve the fatherland.

The Judaeo-Christian cultural community

Suicide was rare among the Jews. In the Old Testament, life was considered to be sacred. A Jew was allowed to break religious laws to save his life, but he must not commit murder, deny God or practise incest. Suicide was regarded in Jewish law as a wrongful and unworthy act. A suicidal act was punished by the victim and the victim's family being denied the usual burial and mourning ritual. In extreme circumstances, however, suicide could be accepted. This was the case, for example, if disgrace could be avoided through suicide in the event of captivity or torture.

Four suicides are described in the Old Testament: Samson, Saul, Abimelech and Achitophael. Samson killed himself and the Philistines by breaking down the pillars of the temple. Saul killed himself after suffering defeat in battle in order to avoid the disgrace of surrender. Abimelech killed himself after he had been mortally wounded by a woman and did not want the disgrace of having been killed by a woman hanging over him. Finally, Achitophael hanged himself when he failed to betray David to Absalom. An increasing number of suicides was reported in Talmud with a distinct attitude of denunciation.

The early Christian period

Acts of martyrdom were common in the early Christian period. The number of suicides increased during this period, many wishing to come closer to God and Christ and live there for ever. There was a certain pessimistic attitude towards life and a corresponding yearning for the values of eternity. It was not until some time later in the history of Christianity that suicide was prohibited. Augustine wrote his great work, *the State of God*, with the first codification of the Church's displeasure with and denunciation of the fact that suicide was spreading. Life is a gift from God. Breaking with life means committing an unavoidable sin against God and his dominion over life and death. Augustine also denounced suicide committed by women after being raped. Someone taking her own life in this way was just as guilty as the man who had committed the injustice. Augustine's attitude was therefore that suicide is murder, but an exception can be allowed: if there is an absolute commandment from God. A true and noble soul will bear suffering, as Job did. He withstood terrible suffering without depriving himself of life. A person committing suicide dies as the worst sinner.

Suicide was denounced at the Synod in Arles in AD 452 on the basis of the view that 'he who kills himself kills an innocent person and commits murder'. A strongly denunciatory attitude towards suicide gradually developed in Christianity, leading for example to Judas Iscariot's betrayal of Christ for a time being regarded as a lesser sin than the suicide he later committed by hanging himself. At the Synod in Braga in AD 563 it was decided that no religious rituals should be held after suicide. However, in practice the situation gradually developed that suicide was allowed under the following three circumstances: voluntary martyrdom, self-inflicted death through ascestism, and the suicide of the virgin and the married woman to preserve their virtue.

A system of restrictions on the condemnation of suicide was established for the first time at the Synod in Antisidor in AD 590. The Synod at Nîmes in 1096 adopted the resolution that those who committed suicide should be denied the right to be buried in consecrated soil. The situation *NB* gradually developed that the body of the person who had committed suicide was buried outside the churchyard or alongside the churchyard wall. In many parts of Europe the body was dragged through the streets and buried at a crossroads, with a stake driven through it and with a stone placed over the face. Remarkable customs developed, such as in Danzig, where the body of a person who had committed suicide could not be taken out of the house through the door but had to be removed through the   window. If there was no window, a hole had to be knocked through the wall.

The Middle Ages

The same attitudes were expressed throughout most of the Middle Ages. This did not prevent many suicides occurring. On a few occasions, mass suicide occurred in connection with persecution and suppression, such as among the persecuted Albigensians in southern France, where no less than 5000 killed themselves. There were also pogroms against the Jews, for example in England, especially under Richard the Lion-Heart. Six hundred took their own lives in York in 1190 rather than suffer suppression. One of those who unsuccessfully attempted suicide was Joan of Arc, who made the attempt while she was in prison in Beauvoir. When she was brought before the court, the bishops used her attempted suicide as further proof of her alliance with the Devil. In the thirteenth century Thomas Aquinas expressed the official Christian view at this time in his *Summa Theologica* – suicide was absolutely wrong for the following reasons:

(1) It was unnatural.
(2) Every person was a member of a society, and suicide was therefore anti-social.
(3) Life was a gift from God and was not at man's disposal.

It was also around this time that Dante's *Inferno* was written, in which light is shed on attitudes towards suicide at that time. The person who committed suicide was condemned to eternal unrest in the forests of self-destruction in the seventh hell, among heretics and murderers.

The Renaissance and the Reformation brought moderation in the view taken of suicide. Luther's ideas cleared the way for a change from absolutism and subservience to personal decision and personal responsibility. Doubt was cast on what had previously been regarded as absolutes. The view gradually emerged that suicides had to be assessed individually. In his famous book *Anatomy of Melancholy*, Burton (1621) broke emphatically with the church dogmas of the time, and questioned whether suicides were condemned for eternity. Suicide gradually became more accepted in the upper classes of society, but continued to be roundly condemned in the lower classes.

The eighteenth century

Some softening of views on suicide occurred in the eighteenth century. Montesquieu (1721) pointed out that Man is part of Nature, which he has reason to modify, and he also has reason to modify that part of Nature which is in Man himself. Montesquieu sharply criticised the official view of suicide, not least from the point of view of the survivors. Both

Rousseau (1761) and Voltaire (1766) criticised the official view of suicide, whilst Rousseau also romanticised suicide.

One of the most important publications from this period is the *Essay on Suicide* (1783) by the Scottish writer David Hume. This book was so radical that the publisher did not dare to publish it until after Hume's death. Hume argues that it must be Man's right to decide on his own death if pain, illness, shame or poverty make life unbearable. Man does not do anything wrong by committing suicide, but stops doing good. He is fully entitled to avoid evil, including life itself. However, opposing sides continued to argue forcibly against each other. Kant proclaimed the sanctity of life and believed that life must be preserved, whatever the cost might be. On the other hand there was Goethe's *Werters Leiden*, published in 1774. This book swept through Europe and triggered epidemics of suicide. It is a romantic novel influenced by Goethe's own stormy love-affair with the 19-year-old Charlotte Buff and the suicide of one of his closest acquaintances – Jerusalem, the legation secretary – who was unhappily in love with a married woman and shot himself.

Modern times

Schopenhauer stands out in the nineteenth century as the leading writer on suicide. He has incorrectly been regarded as a spokesman for suicide. Schopenhauer was pre-occupied with the suffering of life. He was heavily influenced by eastern philosophy. However, he considered suicide to be a mistake or a foolish act – it was not a true liberation from the suffering life presents. But he opposed the view that suicide is to be considered a crime or a sin – Man has the clear right to take his own life, and he criticised the sanctions imposed by the Church. He was quite emphatic that the person who committed suicide did not seek death because he wanted to take his own life, but because he was not satisfied with the conditions under which he lived. In many ways Schopenhauer anticipated modern psychiatric views on suicide.

In the nineteenth century, suicide came to be increasingly regarded more as a 'shame' than as a sin or crime, as it had been previously. This was the century of strong family ties, the century of the middle class, when it was important for the family to maintain its status in society. Suicide gradually came to be denied, it was considered to be a family secret and was increasingly classified with mental illness. Nietzsche (1844–1900) believed that the individual had a complete moral right to take his own life. He used the expression *Freitot* in *Zarathustra* as synonymous with suicide. One must die at the right time.

More scientific writings on suicide started to appear in the nineteenth century. Psychiatry came under medical influence from around 1800. Founders of schools of psychiatry, such as Esquirol (1838), stressed that virtually all who committed suicide were in fact mentally ill (*La maladie mentale*). At the beginning of this century the greatest systematician in psychiatry, Emil Kraepelin, claimed that only some 30% showed manifest symptoms of mental illness.

Durkheim's book *Le Suicide* (1897) was one of the most important books to be written on this subject. Durkheim stressed that there were three main types of suicide, each of which referred back to a particular disparity between the person committing suicide and the social grouping he lived in. One form of suicide occurred when the life of the person who committed suicide had been too much cut off from society and his will had therefore been broken. He termed this form *egoistic suicide*. The characteristic feature of another form was that the person who committed suicide was too strongly integrated into society and was too strongly identified with society, so that he obliterated himself for its sake. He termed this form of suicide *altruistic suicide*. The characteristic feature of the third form was that the person committing suicide had succumbed to the lack of norms in the society of which he formed part. He called this form of suicide *anomic suicide*. His teachings are still highly respected. He demonstrated clearly the relationship between the individual act which suicide represents and the society the person concerned lives in. Where social solidarity is strong, the tendency towards suicide will be low. Where the feeling of solidarity is weak, suicide will be more common.

Views of suicide in Norway

In the period before Christianity was introduced into Norway, it appears that suicide could be accepted in order to avoid disgrace or painful illnesses, and also when bondsmen followed their masters into death. The first Norwegian laws suggest that there were distinct views on suicide. The Gulating Law states that: 'It is such that each person who dies shall be carried to the church and buried in sacred soil, apart from miscreants, those who betray the King, and murderers, thieves and those who take their own lives. Those who have just been named shall be buried in the tide, where the sea and the green turf meet.'

The oldest Christian laws contain provisions that evil-doers are not to be buried in consecrated soil, and those who commit suicide are mentioned among these evil-doers. In Magnus Lagabøter's National Law, which was in force from 1274 to 1688, suicide is mentioned as an *irreparable deed*. 'If a man kills his own wife or the wife her husband, when the killer has fornicated or intended to fornicate, it is an irreparable deed. This is also the case if someone takes his own life. This is an irreparable deed.'

In Norway suicides in the Middle Ages were often buried among executed criminals or out in the forests. During the eighteenth century in the Nordic countries suicide was regarded just as seriously as killing. It was commonly believed that it would be particularly difficult for people who had taken their own lives (or those of others) to find peace in the next world, and that they would therefore have to return as ghosts who could cause problems for those of the living on whom they wanted to take revenge.

3

Suicide in art

It is tempting to tackle an analysis of the place of suicide in Norwegian literature, however, only a brief summary of suicide in the works of Ibsen will be given here. Ibsen has several suicides among his characters.

Hedda Gabler shot herself in the head whilst her husband Jørgen Tesman, Mrs Elvsted and Judge Brack were nearby. She had suffered many disappointments, not least in connection with her ambitions for her husband to be appointed professor. In many ways her suicide is a *dependency loss suicide* in a socially isolated and frustrated woman who did not want to see her image of herself disturbed. In the same play Løvberg probably also commits suicide, an isolated and frustrated man who over the course of time has slipped out of his relationships and has also developed an alcohol problem.

Another well known suicide is that of Hedvig in *Hedda Gabler*. The young girl, socially isolated in a very special world, strongly attached to her father, could not live with her father's rejection when it dawned on him that she was not his daughter. Social isolation and the loss of an *important other person* are central themes here. In *Rosmersholm* there are no less than three cases of suicide: Johannes' wife in frustration over Rebecca entering his life, later Johannes himself when he becomes aware of the role he played in her death, and Rebecca who fell into the waterfall with him.

Other suicides that can be mentioned are that of Hjørdis in *The Vikings at Helgeland*, again committed in frustration over the fact that she had to marry someone else rather than the one she thought she had the right to marry. Her plan was to kill the one she loved, Sigurd, and at the same time kill herself so that they could live together in death. When he told her that he had become a Christian and that they could not therefore be together after death, she was the one who jumped off the cliff.

Altogether there are seven definite cases of suicide in Ibsen's plays, but the others are more peripheral to the story. There are also a total of five cases of victim-precipitated suicide, including Agathon in *Emperor and Galilean* and Hertug Skule and his son.

Thomas Hjortsjø (1985b) has written a review of suicide in painting. According to him, the following classifications can be made:

- Suicide as a *heroic act*. This category includes *patriotic suicide*, such as Ruben's painting of the Roman consul Decius Mus, who sacrificed his life so that the Romans could overcome their enemies. Suicide carried out to preserve dignity is also placed in this category. Princess Dido committed suicide by burning herself to avoid a marriage she could not accept, and the suicide of Lucretia was a consequence of her being forced into sexual intercourse with Prince Tarquinus Sextus.
- Suicide as a *stigmatising act* is exemplified by the suicide of Nero, detested as he was because of his persecution of the Christians.
- Suicide as an *irrational act* is personified in Delacroix's painting of Ophelia, who became mentally ill after the death of her father.
- Suicide as a *romanticised act* was often portrayed in the nineteenth century, as in the death of the 17-year-old Thomas Chatterton, painted by Wallis.
- Suicide as a *depressive act* is found in Manet's Suicidi, Nettis' I Suicidi and Toulouse-Lautrec's La Pendue. Edvard Munch's The Dead Couple and The Suicide are clear and telling examples of the connection between depression and suicide.
- Suicide as an *ambivalent act* is exemplified in Daumier's L'Imagination, which shows a person pondering over seven apparently unacceptable methods for taking one's own life.
- Suicide as a *cry for help* has also been portrayed, particularly in modern painting, which is oriented more towards social realism (Lebrun, Warhol, Lichtenstein).

Hjortsjø concludes his review of suicide in western painting as follows:

> Classical art which over the centuries often and usually portrays self-chosen death, emphasises the value of life, seen against the background of the life situation of the victim, but also from the point of view of the overriding ethical and religious conceptions which from one period to another have predominated in society. Artists early on became the tool

with which the prevailing attitude could be spread and maintained. By not touching on pathological and taboo areas, artists in earlier times gave suicide a glamorous appearance. The figurative and non-figurative artists of later periods are generally anchored far more strongly in social realism.

Those interested should read two Swedish articles by Thomas Hjortsjø (1985a,b).

4

Incidence – statistical data

Records in most European countries go back to the last century. It is difficult to compare data from different periods of time, and even more difficult to compare data from different countries. There are different ways of recording suicide, and in some cases methods of recording have changed within individual countries. Sources of error in an area may be great in one country and produce data which cannot be readily compared with data from another country. These sources of error may relate to the recording systems but may also be associated with taboos. In most countries it is the doctor who makes the diagnosis of the cause of death, and they will naturally be influenced by the taboos prevailing in their particular country.

The figures are consistently lower in southern European Catholic countries than in northern European Protestant countries. This may relate to the fact that religion is stronger in the southern Catholic countries, that cohesion is consequently stronger, that confession relieves people of some of their problems and feelings of guilt, and that people live in a closer family relationship and in a closer relationship to one another and to religion. It may also, however, relate to the fact that suicide is surrounded by stronger taboos and is the object of greater general moral prejudice in strictly Catholic countries. This may in turn lead those close to the victim to try to a greater extent to conceal the act, out of concern for the unfortunate individual and the family. Doctors are obviously subject to the same taboos as the population at large. However, the differences may just as well relate to the fact that the recording technique is better in northern Protestant countries, and that the traditions associated with recording and reporting procedures are stricter. The possibility that the latter factor may be of significance is suggested by studies from Canada. These show that the suicide rate is just as high in the French-speaking Catholic part as in the predominantly Protestant English-speaking part of the country.

It is difficult to draw conclusions from the differences in suicide rate between countries. In most countries the cause of death is specified by the general practitioner, however, in England suicide is recorded through a coroner, who does not pronounce the verdict of suicide unless there is positive evidence of suicide, for example in the form of a suicide note. Comparing studies, therefore between countries such as England and Denmark has clearly shown that the figures cannot be directly compared.

There are also significant regional differences in suicide rate within an individual country. Differences of this kind usually tie in with population groups. Hungary, for example, has the highest suicide rate in Europe. Countries bordering on Hungary usually have their highest suicide rate in those areas which are close to the border or which have Hungarian minorities. In fact regional differences of this kind have been observed in most countries.

Hungary has topped the suicide statistics in Europe in recent years. The suicide rate there stands at 60 per 100,000 per year. Finland and Denmark are also near the top in Europe, with a suicide rate of around 30. Countries such as Poland, Czechoslovakia, Switzerland, Austria and the former West Germany all have a suicide rate of between 20 and 30 per 100,000 per year (see Table 4.1). Medium-level rates are found for example in Great Britain and Sweden. Norway has been a low suicide country for around 100 years, but has joined the medium-level group over the past 15–20 years, with a rate of around 16. Countries in Europe with a low suicide rate are Italy, Spain, Portugal, Scotland and Ireland in recent years . However, the suicide rate has risen very sharply in Ireland in recent years. Most non-European countries also have a low suicide rate. This applies for example to South America. The USA is in the middle band. The suicide rate in Iceland has been close to that in Norway, whilst it has been markedly lower on the Faeroes. In contrast to these two parts of the Nordic region, Greenland has the highest suicide rate in Europe, approx. 127. The background to this is assumed to be the culture clash between the original Greenland culture and the influence of western culture through Denmark. Greenland characteristically also has a serious alcohol problem and a high incidence of sexually transmitted diseases. Both these factors are assumed to relate to the fact that the traditional norms are being dissipated, whilst no adjustment to the new norms has yet been made.

A significant increase in the suicide rate occurred in all European countries over the ten-year period from 1973 to 1983. The increase was greatest in Ireland, where it was 128% for men and 127% for women. Next comes Northern Ireland, with an increase of 137% and 53%. Regrettably Norway takes third place in these sorry statistics, with an increase of 57% for men and 57% for women. The increase in Denmark was relatively modest, at 18 and 8%, and in Finland there was a slight decline overall, suicide among men having only increased by 1% and among women having fallen by 6%.

A statistical study of what the changes have been like in the younger part of the population in a number of countries unfortunately produces very alarming results as far as Norway is concerned. The number of suicides in the 15–19 age group showed a seven-fold increase over the period from 1970 to 1985. There is only one country in Europe where the increase was greater, namely in Ireland, where there was an eight-fold increase for this age group. The rate in Denmark slightly more than doubled over this period.

There are three countries showing a fall in the suicide rate in this age group. These are countries which traditionally have very high suicide rates: Hungary, Japan and the former West Germany.

The picture is similar for the 20–24 age group. Most countries have a moderate to large increase, Norway a more than doubling and Ireland nearly a three-fold increase. Hungary, Japan and West Germany also reveal a moderate fall in this age group. For the 25–29 age group the situation is slightly different. Here Ireland shows a huge rise, namely a thirteen-fold increase, whilst in Norway there was *only* a doubling.

The development with respect to young people is best illustrated in Figure 4.1, which shows the percentage increase in suicide mortality in 13 countries over the period 1970–1985, for (a) young people aged 15–19, (b) young people aged 20–24 and (c) young people aged 25–29. The source is the WHO data bank (Diekstra, 1989b).

USA and Canada

The suicide rate among young people also increased sharply in the USA during the 1960s and 1970s.

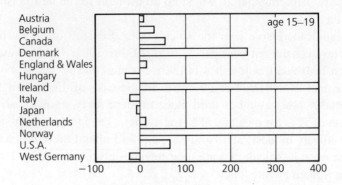

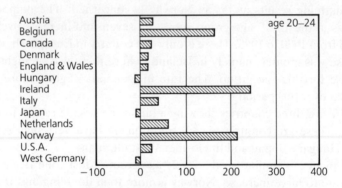

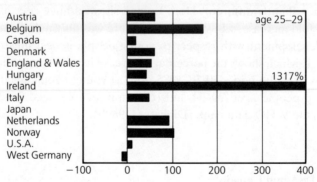

Figure 4.1. Suicide mortality, increase in per cent in 13 countries, 1970–85 (from Diekstra, 1989b).

The increase from 1960 to 1975 was 130% for the 20–24 age group. The problem of violence is greater in the USA than in many other western European countries. The most common cause of death among young adults (age 15–24) is accidents, followed by homicide, with suicide in third place. For teenagers (age 15–19) the rate rose from 3.6 per 100,000 in 1960 to 8.7 per 100,000 in 1981, an increase of 142%. It is the rate for males which increased most over this period, from 5.6 to 13.6 per 100,000. The increase was greater for whites than for blacks. The rise in the total suicide rate for all ages was due particularly to the increase among young men. The official figures for 1986 show that the suicide rate for the 15–24 age group was 13.1 per 100,000, which corresponds to 5120 suicides per year in this ten-year age group – the equivalent of 14 suicides per day. Suicide accounted for 12.8% of the deaths in this age group.

In many countries an increase is occurring in the suicide rate among the 13–14 age group. The suicide rate for the 10–14 age group is usually low. However, it too has increased in recent years, and in the USA it now stands at just under one per 100,000. In 1981 there were 167 suicides in the 5–14 age group in the USA, and only four of these were under the age of 10. The suicide rate varies greatly between states in the USA. In Alaska, for example, the suicide rate for the 15–24 age group in 1978 was 25.4 per 100,000 (Seiden, 1984), but in New Jersey it was as low as 6.5 per 100,000. In Canada there is an increase in suicide among young people – the suicide rate for young men in Alberta has increased 12 to 15 times since 1950, and a similar development has taken place in Ontario (Garfinkel & Golombek, 1983).

How the suicide rate in the USA among men in the 15–24 age group developed in relation to the rate for the population as a whole from 1900 through to the 1980s can be seen in Figure 4.2, taken from Hendin (1982).

Suicide among the elderly has also shown a clear increase in the USA. Those over the age of 50 constituted 26% of the total population of the USA in 1980, but accounted for 39% of all deaths from suicide. If only the white section of the population over the age of 50 is looked at, representing 23% of the population, 37% of those who commit suicide are from this group. Even more clearly, white men over the age of 50 make up 10% of the population but account for 28% of all deaths from suicide (Hendin, 1982). Hendin states that three-quarters of all suicides among those over the age of 50 are committed by men, and 96% of these male suicides are carried out by white males.

Rate per 100,000 Population

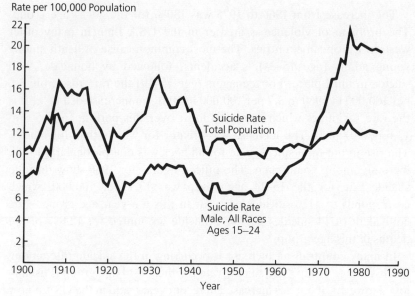

Figure 4.2. US suicide rates total population and males 15–24 (from Hendin, 1982).

What factors can be put forward to explain these trends?

Sainsbury, Jenkins & Levey (1982) in co-operation with the WHO studied the relationship between changes in social conditions and changes in suicide rate after 1960 in 18 European countries. The social characteristics in countries which in 1961–63 could foresee a subsequent rise in the suicide rate were:

(1) A high divorce rate which can be regarded as an expression of the trend towards alienation in society.
(2) A low percentage of the population below the age of 15, which points to the extent to which people live outside of family groups.
(3) A high unemployment rate.
(4) A high murder rate.

In addition, Sainsbury found a high number of women in working life among whom the rate of suicide was increasing, which may reflect changes in status and also an increased stress factor for women. Factors (1), (2) and (3) may also indicate changes in the family structure within society.

Sainsbury *et al.* (1982) in the same paper analyse changes in social conditions after 1960 and how these related to changes in the national suicide rates. The results were similar to those just mentioned, but not entirely identical. An increased suicide rate was linked to:

(1) A decline in the population under the age of 15.
(2) An increase in the percentage of the population over the age of 65, that is the age group which has traditionally had the highest suicide rate in the European countries.
(3) An increase in the 'third period of training' for women. The entry of women into the working world, possibly also an indicator of changes both in the status of women and in family structure.

There were two further indicators which stood out with regard to the increase in suicide rates:

(4) An increase in alcohol consumption showed a strong correlation with an increase in the suicide rate.
(5) A link between increased suicide rate and a decline in religious commitment and church activities, which is probably reflected in moral values and attitudes towards suicide, and also suggests declining social integration. The church has over the centuries acted as a social network for people.

To summarise, it can be said that the studies referred to here suggest that societies and social groups which are exposed to economic instability and unemployment, the breakdown of traditional values in the primary family and in groups, increasing violence and criminal behaviour, secularisation and increased abuse of alcohol and drugs are highly prone to having increased suicide rates, and rates which are higher than they were previously in the society in question. An increase in suicide rates can, therefore, be expected among the young and also in what are referred to as the developing countries over the next decade, since it may be assumed that traditional values will also break down there.

Figure 4.3 shows the percentage change in the suicide rate from 1960–61 to 1984–85 (Diekstra, 1989b). This diagram shows the overall figures for both sexes and all ages.

Finally Table 4.1 shows the changes in the suicide rate per 100,000 among those over the age of 15 in 24 European countries, classified according to sex (the average for 1972–73 compared with the average for 1983–84).

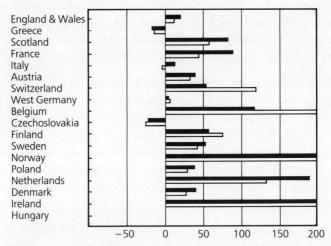

Figure 4.3. Percentage change in suicide rate 1960–61 and 1984–85, both sexes and all ages (from Diekstra, 1989b); darks bars = observed change, light bars = predicted change.

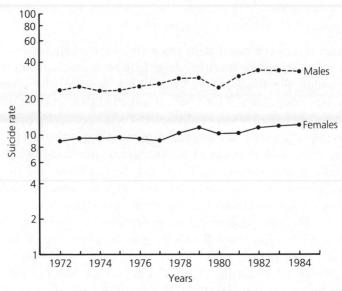

Figure 4.4. The median rate is based on 24 countries in 1972–74, 1978 and 1979; on 23 countries in 1975–77 and 1980; on 22 countries in 1983; and on 21 countries in 1981, 1982 and 1984 (from Platt, 1989).

Table 4.1. *Changes in the suicide rate per 100,000 in those aged 15 and over in 24 European countries according to sex (average 1972–73 to average 1983–84)*

Country	Men			Women		
	av. 1972–73	av. 1983–84	change (%)	av. 1972–73	av. 1983–84	change (%)
Austria	43.7	50.1	+14.6	18.1	18.2	+0.6
Belgium	27.8	39.2	+41.0	12.6	19.0	+50.8
Bulgaria	20.6	28.0	+35.9	8.9	10.6	+19.1
Czechoslovakia	45.6	38.7	−15.1	16.0	12.2	−23.8
Denmark	38.8	45.7	+17.8	23.5	25.3	+7.7
Finland	50.5	51.0	+1.0	13.0	12.2	−6.2
France	30.3	41.3	+36.3	11.6	15.4	+32.8
FRG	35.2	34.5	−2.0	18.2	16.1	−11.5
Greece	5.4	7.2	+33.3	2.3	2.6	+13.0
Hungary	67.4	86.9	+28.9	26.5	32.7	+23.4
Iceland	23.4	38.9	+66.2	8.4	8.0	−4.8
Ireland	6.8	15.5	+127.9	2.6	5.9	+126.9
Italy	10.9	12.9	+18.3	4.6	5.5	+19.6
Luxembourg	25.2	36.7	+45.6	11.0	14.1	+28.2
Netherlands	13.5	18.7	+38.5	9.4	11.8	+25.5
Norway	17.3	27.2	+57.2	6.1	9.6	+57.4
Poland	26.7	29.9	+12.0	5.5	6.0	+9.1
Portugal	19.0	19.5	+2.6	5.2	7.1	+36.5
Spain	8.9	8.9	–	3.1	2.9	−6.5
Sweden	37.4	33.8	−9.6	14.6	13.8	−5.5
Switzerland	36.6	44.6	+21.9	14.0	16.9	+20.7
United Kingdom						
– England and Wales	12.4	14.7	+18.5	8.0	7.0	−12.5
– Northern Ireland	5.9	14.0	+137.3	4.9	7.5	+53.1
– Scotland	13.5	18.0	+33.3	8.9	7.4	−16.9

Note: (From Diekstra, 1989b.)

In addition to mentioning the changes which have been examined here, reference must be made to a survey carried out by Platt of suicide trends in 24 European countries over the period 1972–84 (Platt, 1989; Figure 4.4). Platt emphasises his view, with which I agree, that although it is possible to discuss comparisons between countries, there are many sources of error that need to be considered, whilst the development over time within the same country probably produces a relatively relevant comparison. The analyses Platt gives are taken from the WHO (Tables 4.2, 4.3).

Table 4.2. Crude suicide rate per 100,000 males aged 15+ years in 24 european countries, 1972–84[a]

Country	1972	1973	1974	1975	1976	1977	1978	1979	1980	1981	1982	1983	1984
Austria	44.9	42.5	45.2	47.4	43.6	45.3	47.2	47.2	47.8	51.3	53.2	50.1	50.1
Belgium	28.2	27.3	28.1	27.4	28.4	32.0	34.8	35.6	36.0	37.0	37.6	37.7	40.7
Bulgaria	20.5	20.7	22.8	23.4	25.5	26.6	24.7	25.7	24.5	24.7	27.9	24.9	31.0
Czechoslovakia	47.1	44.0	44.9	42.6	40.8	43.2	42.4	40.1	39.8	40.6	40.2	39.6	37.7
Denmark	39.4	38.2	44.0	38.8	39.2	39.9	36.0	40.7	52.4	49.0	46.4	46.1	45.3
Finland	51.6	49.4	53.1	52.6	54.7	54.0	53.7	51.7	52.9	49.2	48.5	50.1	51.9
France	30.7	29.9	29.9	30.0	29.8	30.3	32.0	35.0	35.9	36.5	38.9	40.6	41.9
FRG	34.5	35.8	36.2	35.8	37.2	38.3	37.7	36.1	34.9	36.1	36.1	34.8	34.1
Greece	5.3	5.4	6.1	4.6	5.0	6.2	5.5	5.3	6.0	6.1	6.5	6.9	7.4
Hungary	67.6	67.1	74.5	70.7	73.9	71.6	77.5	82.1	83.1	82.3	80.7	86.5	87.3
Iceland	16.7	30.0	21.3	18.3	17.9	22.8	28.7	30.6	16.9	14.3	17.5	36.8	41.0
Ireland	6.3	7.3	8.7	9.7	11.6	8.6	9.2	12.3	11.9	13.2	14.6	16.4	NA
Italy	10.9	10.8	9.8	10.4	10.5	11.7	12.2	12.8	13.1	12.7	NA	NA	NA
Luxembourg	26.2	24.2	23.5	NA	NA	NA	34.7	34.0	24.5	31.4	41.7	40.9	32.5
Netherlands	13.7	13.3	14.8	14.5	15.8	15.2	14.5	15.4	16.6	15.6	16.6	18.4	19.0
Norway	17.2	17.3	21.5	18.6	21.1	22.2	22.7	22.5	23.4	24.6	26.2	26.7	27.6
Poland	27.2	26.1	24.7	25.6	27.1	27.8	30.0	28.8	NA	NA	NA	28.0	31.8
Portugal	18.9	19.1	18.5	18.9	19.6	19.5	20.1	21.2	15.5	15.5	16.4	19.5	19.4
Spain	9.2	8.5	7.9	8.3	8.4	8.4	8.3	8.5	9.2	NA	NA	NA	NA
Sweden	37.3	37.4	36.4	35.2	33.6	35.9	33.1	35.6	34.5	30.7	34.5	33.7	33.8
Switzerland	37.0	35.9	38.1	42.4	41.5	43.7	43.7	43.7	46.0	42.0	43.4	45.1	44.0
UK – England and Wales	12.3	12.5	12.6	12.0	12.8	12.9	13.2	13.8	14.0	14.5	14.6	14.6	14.8
UK – Northern Ireland	5.9	5.8	7.3	6.8	7.9	7.1	7.0	9.9	9.8	NA	10.0	15.3	12.8
UK – Scotland	13.1	13.8	14.1	12.1	13.3	13.1	14.5	15.2	16.8	17.7	18.8	17.6	18.3

Note: NA, not available.
[a] Source: WHO data bank.
Source: (From Platt, 1989.)

Table 4.3. *Crude suicide rate per 100,000 females aged 15+ years in 24 European countries, 1972–84[a]*

Country	1972	1973	1974	1975	1976	1977	1978	1979	1980	1981	1982	1983	1984
Austria	18.6	17.5	18.5	17.6	17.0	18.8	17.8	18.2	18.3	18.4	17.5	18.6	17.8
Belgium	13.0	11.9	13.0	14.6	14.4	16.8	17.6	18.6	19.8	18.3	17.1	19.3	18.7
Bulgaria	8.8	8.9	9.7	9.5	10.4	10.2	10.0	11.2	10.3	10.1	11.0	9.2	11.9
Czechoslovakia	17.1	14.8	15.4	15.1	14.5	13.6	14.9	13.1	13.8	12.8	13.3	12.1	12.2
Denmark	22.8	23.8	23.6	23.6	22.6	22.6	23.7	24.9	27.9	26.5	26.1	24.9	25.7
Finland	12.8	13.1	13.3	13.2	12.9	13.3	12.0	12.1	13.2	11.9	13.0	12.1	12.3
France	12.0	11.2	11.3	11.5	11.5	12.6	12.6	13.4	13.9	13.9	14.7	15.3	15.4
FRG	17.8	18.5	18.5	18.2	18.5	19.5	18.4	17.6	16.9	17.2	16.0	16.7	15.4
Greece	2.0	2.5	3.1	2.6	2.3	2.6	2.0	2.4	2.4	2.6	2.6	2.5	2.7
Hungary	26.4	26.5	28.9	27.2	30.2	31.7	33.5	33.4	33.2	36.1	32.9	33.1	32.2
Iceland	8.4	8.3	8.1	10.6	5.2	5.1	3.7	4.9	12.1	4.8	8.2	8.1	7.9
Ireland	2.4	2.7	2.4	4.1	4.8	4.7	4.9	4.1	6.1	5.4	5.2	6.5	NA
Italy	4.7	4.4	4.5	4.4	4.5	4.8	4.8	5.4	5.8	5.1	NA	NA	NA
Luxembourg	12.1	9.8	9.0	NA	NA	NA	11.5	16.6	7.9	10.4	11.6	14.1	14.0
Netherlands	8.7	10.0	9.9	9.3	9.3	9.0	10.7	11.7	9.5	10.0	10.6	11.7	11.9
Norway	6.6	5.5	5.9	7.2	7.3	7.6	7.7	9.1	8.4	8.3	9.4	10.2	8.9
Poland	5.4	5.6	5.4	4.8	5.2	5.2	5.4	5.2	NA	NA	NA	5.6	6.4
Portugal	4.8	5.5	5.8	5.5	5.0	5.9	6.4	6.3	5.0	5.9	6.2	6.6	7.5
Spain	3.1	3.1	3.0	2.7	2.9	2.9	2.9	2.8	2.9	NA	NA	NA	NA
Sweden	14.1	15.1	14.4	13.8	14.1	14.0	14.7	16.0	13.9	13.0	13.7	13.2	14.3
Switzerland	14.4	13.6	15.9	16.4	15.9	17.9	17.8	19.1	18.6	17.6	17.7	16.9	16.8
UK – England and Wales	8.0	8.0	8.2	7.6	7.5	7.9	7.9	8.1	8.3	8.1	7.2	7.0	7.0
UK – Northern Ireland	2.9	6.8	4.1	3.6	4.6	5.6	5.6	3.8	4.6	NA	6.0	8.9	6.1
UK – Scotland	8.9	8.8	8.5	9.6	8.7	8.4	7.8	9.5	9.2	8.2	9.1	7.5	7.3

Note: NA, not available.
[a] Source: WHO data bank.
Source: (From Platt, 1989.)

Table 4.4. *Ratio of male:female suicide rate (per 100,000 population aged 15+ years) in 24 European countries, 1972–73 and 1983–84[a,b]*

Country	M:F ratio	
	1972–73	1983–84[a]
Austria	2.4	2.8
Belgium	2.2	2.1
Bulgaria	2.3	2.6
Czechoslovakia	2.9	3.2
Denmark	1.7	1.8
Finland	3.9	4.2
France	2.6	2.7
FRG	1.9	2.1
Greece	2.3	2.8
Hungary	2.5	2.7
Iceland	2.8	4.9
Ireland	2.6	2.6
Italy	2.4	2.3
Luxembourg	2.3	2.6
Netherlands	1.4	1.6
Norway	2.8	2.8
Poland	4.9	5.0
Portugal	3.7	2.7
Spain	2.9	3.1
Sweden	2.6	2.4
Switzerland	2.6	2.6
United Kingdom		
– England and Wales	1.6	2.1
– Northern Ireland	1.2	1.9
– Scotland	1.5	2.4

Note: [a] Except for the following countries (latest years in parentheses): Ireland (1982–83), Italy (1980–81), Spain (1979–80).
[b] Source: WHO data bank.
Source: (From Platt, 1989.)

The ratio between men and women has also been assessed and can be seen in Table 4.4.

It is important to note from this table that the ratio between men and women was higher in the last period than in the first in 17 countries, and that there were only four countries where the ratio was lower. It thus appears that on a European basis there is a greater preponderance of men, a surprising trend since the pattern of roles for the sexes is in the process of narrowing.

Table 4.5. *Age-specific suicide rate per 100,000 males in 24 European countries, mean 1983–84[a,b]*

Country	Age groups						
	15–24	25–34	35–44	45–54	55–64	65–74	75+
Austria	30.2	37.3	52.6	60.3	52.5	71.4	105.6
Belgium	16.0	36.9	37.1	39.8	44.6	60.8	94.6
Bulgaria	10.2	19.8	22.7	26.0	34.9	53.6	108.0
Czechoslovakia	14.8	31.1	38.3	48.1	43.4	62.6	100.1
Denmark	15.7	36.5	52.0	58.7	63.7	53.0	75.4
Finland	36.3	53.9	53.4	60.4	52.2	53.6	55.8
France	16.4	33.2	36.8	43.4	46.7	64.5	114.6
FRG	19.4	28.3	33.7	40.1	38.1	48.9	73.5
Greece	4.9	7.0	5.1	6.2	9.8	9.3	14.8
Hungary	26.8	60.5	96.3	115.0	102.8	123.8	190.6
Iceland	(37.9)	(20.1)	(35.9)	(46.2)	(41.9)	(94.6)	(34.9)
Ireland	12.4	17.7	15.7	13.6	19.3	19.1	(11.4)
Italy	5.2	8.3	9.0	14.0	16.8	25.7	36.9
Luxembourg	(19.4)	(37.0)	(38.7)	(37.3)	(41.2)	(45.1)	(73.8)
Netherlands	7.3	17.9	17.9	20.6	25.2	27.9	45.7
Norway	23.4	23.8	21.5	33.2	38.4	29.3	25.1
Poland	18.5	34.0	34.2	36.0	30.0	27.3	26.8
Portugal	10.3	14.0	16.6	20.7	29.5	32.7	42.5
Spain	4.2	5.3	6.5	9.8	12.3	17.0	30.5
Sweden	16.3	34.0	34.4	43.4	32.8	39.7	50.7
Switzerland	33.7	39.5	40.2	48.8	51.4	59.6	64.8
United Kingdom							
– England and Wales	7.1	14.0	16.3	17.8	17.5	17.3	22.5
– Northern Ireland	(9.2)	(12.4)	(15.2)	(12.9)	(16.4)	(18.0)	(18.8)
– Scotland	9.7	17.7	20.2	24.5	21.3	20.3	(18.1)

Note: Rate in parentheses based on mean of <20 suicides per annum
[a] Except for the following countries (latest years in parentheses): Ireland (1982–83), Italy (1980–81), Spain (1979–80).
[b] Source: WHO data bank.
Source: (From Platt, 1989.)

It can be seen from Tables 4.5 and 4.6 that there is a rising rate with age, with a peak around the age of 75. There are only four countries which have markedly differing patterns: Finland and Norway, where there is no clear age-related trend, and Poland and Scotland, with a peak in the 45–54 age group. Ten of the 24 countries showed a peak in this age group in 1983–84, compared with only three in 1972–73. Changes in the age-specific suicide rates for men and women in the period are given in Tables 4.7, 4.8 and 4.9.

Table 4.6. *Age-specific suicide rate per 100,000 females in 24 European countries, mean 1983–84[a,b]*

Country	Age groups 15–24	25–34	35–44	45–54	55–64	65–74	75+
Austria	8.2	9.5	15.0	22.2	21.7	28.2	35.0
Belgium	4.1	12.8	18.5	26.5	27.7	27.9	25.7
Bulgaria	4.6	4.2	5.4	8.3	13.8	24.0	37.3
Czechoslovakia	4.1	7.2	7.6	12.8	16.1	21.9	34.9
Denmark	(4.7)	14.4	26.4	36.7	39.5	37.6	32.5
Finland	5.8	12.4	12.2	17.1	15.3	12.6	11.6
France	4.7	11.2	13.3	16.9	19.7	25.1	(28.8)
FRG	5.8	9.7	14.1	17.3	21.1	25.6	27.8
Greece	(2.1)	(2.2)	(1.4)	3.4	(2.8)	(3.9)	(3.6)
Hungary	8.4	16.6	29.9	33.6	39.4	54.1	81.0
Iceland	(0)	(5.4)	(22.5)	(13.9)	(10.3)	(7.0)	(0)
Ireland	(2.7)	(3.9)	(7.1)	(8.0)	(12.7)	(6.4)	(3.2)
Italy	2.1	3.2	4.3	6.0	8.0	9.9	9.0
Luxembourg	(7.1)	(13.8)	(12.4)	(23.6)	(14.0)	(15.0)	(15.5)
Netherlands	3.5	9.8	10.6	15.6	17.3	20.2	16.4
Norway	(4.3)	(6.2)	10.3	15.1	16.1	11.2	(6.7)
Poland	4.2	5.6	5.8	7.4	7.0	7.2	6.3
Portugal	5.6	4.7	5.8	8.3	6.3	13.3	9.6
Spain	1.2	1.2	2.2	3.4	4.3	5.0	6.2
Sweden	6.2	13.5	14.9	19.6	15.5	16.5	11.8
Switzerland	7.9	12.6	16.6	20.8	22.2	23.7	21.4
United Kingdom							
– England and Wales	1.9	3.6	6.4	9.5	10.7	11.1	10.0
– Northern Ireland	(3.0)	(6.7)	(8.0)	(7.5)	(16.3)	(7.5)	(6.4)
– Scotland	(1.9)	(5.5)	8.5	9.3	11.5	11.1	(7.2)

Note: Rate in parentheses based on mean of <20 suicides per annum
[a] Except for the following countries (latest years in parentheses): Ireland (1982–83), Italy (1980–81), Spain (1979–80).
[b] Source: WHO data bank.
Source: (From Platt, 1989.)

Platt states that two findings from the age-specific trends merit attention. The first of these is what is known as the 'Twin Peak Profile'. Although the suicide rates continue to show a direct connection with age, most countries now report a peak in younger age groups (45–54) than previously. The other finding is the trend towards those in the 25–34 age group showing the greatest increase in suicide rate in the period under discussion. There has been great concern in the USA over an epidemic of suicide among teenagers and young adults (in the 15–24 age group), and

Table 4.7. *Changes in age-specific suicide rate per 100,000 males in 24 European countries, mean 1972–73 to mean 1983–84[a],[b]*

Country	Age groups (%)						
	15–24	25–34	35–44	45–54	55–64	65–74	75+
Austria	+52.5	+27.3	+27.1	+17.1	−20.6	+11.7	+21.9
Belgium	+53.8	+26.9	+91.2	+49.6	+12.3	+0.1	+8.4
Bulgaria	+8.5	+81.7	+61.0	+43.6	+34.7	+9.4	+9.2
Czechoslovakia	−48.1	−10.1	−20.7	−8.6	−15.7	−5.2	−2.7
Denmark	+25.6	+50.2	+16.1	+8.3	+9.3	+4.1	+23.8
Finland	+13.4	+18.7	−2.2	−5.0	−23.5	−11.0	−16.2
France	+113.0	+174.4	+109.1	+74.3	+53.1	+82.2	+185.1
FRG	−6.3	+7.2	−2.3	−2.4	−17.0	−2.2	+15.4
Greece	(+96.0)	+89.2	(+70.0)	+19.2	+16.7	−14.7	0
Hungary	+4.7	+25.5	+40.8	+33.7	+12.7	+20.8	+16.1
Iceland	(+161.4)	(+36.7)	(−17.8)	(+139.4)	(−6.1)	(+240.3)	(−)
Ireland	(+287.5)	(+168.2)	(+153.2)	(+70.0)	(+82.1)	(+103.2)	(+50.0)
Italy	+33.3	+40.7	+15.4	+28.4	−1.2	+3.6	+5.1
Luxembourg	(+921.1)	(+141.8)	(+43.3)	(+51.6)	(+32.9)	(−26.2)	(+1.0)
Netherlands	+17.7	+126.6	+46.7	+29.6	+16.7	+17.2	+23.8
Norway	+136.4	+84.5	+32.7	+32.3	+64.8	+42.9	(+42.6)
Poland	−1.6	+30.8	+11.8	+9.4	−10.2	0	−3.6
Portugal	+134.1	+75.0	+13.7	−9.2	−7.5	−23.2	−41.1
Spain	+82.6	+29.3	−4.4	−6.7	−15.2	−25.1	+7.8
Sweden	−10.4	+8.6	−18.5	−7.3	−29.6	−5.5	+4.3
Switzerland	+48.5	+52.5	+16.9	+22.9	+1.2	+7.8	−10.2
United Kingdom							
– England and Wales	+18.3	+44.3	+33.6	+29.0	+10.1	−8.9	+9.2
– N. Ireland	(+162.9)	(+287.5)	(+108.2)	(+121.0)	(+27.1)	(+462.5)	(+683.3)
– Scotland	+20.0	+68.6	+44.3	+57.1	+17.7	+10.9	(+16.0)

Note: Rate in parentheses based on mean of <20 suicides per annum in one or both time periods
[a] Except for the following countries (latest years in parentheses): Ireland (1982–83), Italy (1980–81), Spain (1979–80).
[b] Source: WHO data bank.
Source: (From Platt, 1989.)

Table 4.8. *Changes in age-specific suicide rate per 100,000 females in 24 European countries, mean 1972–73 to 1983–84[a,b]*

Country	Age groups (%)						
	15–24	25–34	35–44	45–54	55–64	65–74	75+
Austria	+34.4	+3.3	+15.4	−3.5	−13.2	+8.0	+6.1
Belgium	+5.1	+77.8	+112.6	+94.9	+45.0	+18.7	+27.2
Bulgaria	+17.9	+20.0	+38.5	+6.4	−14.3	+20.0	+18.4
Czechoslovakia	−48.8	−20.9	−37.7	−21.5	−19.9	−20.7	−20.1
Denmark	(−24.2)	+110.8	+15.3	+3.1	−0.3	+9.9	+67.5
Finland	−31.0	+12.7	−12.2	+8.2	−19.9	−10.0	(+24.7)
France	+6.8	+67.2	+56.5	+28.0	+15.9	+23.6	(+41.9)
FRG	−13.4	−10.2	−2.1	−23.8	−20.7	−1.9	+1.1
Greece	(+40.0)	(+100.0)	(−17.6)	(+70.0)	(−17.6)	(−4.9)	(−21.7)
Hungary	+18.3	+21.2	+51.0	+6.7	+11.3	+7.3	+20.7
Iceland	(−)	(−64.7)	(+150.0)	(+183.7)	(−44.3)	(−)	(−)
Ireland	(+125.0)	(+85.7)	(+163.0)	(+48.1)	(+353.6)	(+137.0)	(+128.6)
Italy	+5.0	+14.3	+22.9	+20.0	+8.1	+23.8	+25.0
Luxembourg	(+82.1)	(+115.6)	(+195.2)	(+80.2)	(−38.6)	(−25.4)	(+37.2)
Netherlands	+12.9	+55.6	+17.8	+19.1	+12.3	+37.4	+28.1
Norway	(+13.2)	(+21.6)	+77.6	+62.4	(+94.0)	(+75.0)	(+91.4)
Poland	+7.7	+24.4	+1.8	+1.4	0	+7.5	+16.7
Portugal	(+124.0)	(+30.6)	+65.7	+43.1	−18.2	+46.2	(−13.5)
Spain	+50.0	−14.3	0	−17.1	−15.7	−18.0	−6.1
Sweden	−27.1	+19.5	−5.1	−1.0	−22.5	+7.1	+6.3
Switzerland	+27.4	+17.8	+37.2	+6.7	+11.0	+42.8	−4.9
United Kingdom							
– England and Wales	−63.3	−25.0	−12.3	−9.5	−5.3	−2.6	−5.7
– N. Ireland	(+130.8)	(+148.1)	(+21.2)	(+63.0)	(+79.1)	(−21.9)	(+357.1)
– Scotland	(−5.0)	(+20.3)	+2.4	−15.5	−27.7	+5.7	(−28.7)

Note: Rate in parentheses based on mean of <20 suicides per annum in one or both time periods.
[a] Except for the following countries (latest years in parentheses): Ireland (1982–82), Italy (1980–81), Spain (1979–80),

Table 4.9. *Summary of changes in age-specific suicide rates, 1972–73 to 1983–84*

Age group	Median change (%)	Range of change (%)	Overall change over period			
			Increase (no. of countries)	Decrease (no. of countries)	Same (no. of countries)	Significance[a]
Males[b]						
15–24 years	+22.8	−48.1 to +136.4	16	4	0	$P = .012$
25–34 years	+42.5	−10.1 to +174.4	19	1	0	$P < .001$
35–44 years	+22.0	−20.7 to +109.1	15	5	0	$P = .042$
45–54 years	+21.1	−9.2 to +74.3	14	6	0	NS
55–64 years	+5.3	−29.6 to +64.8	11	9	0	NS
65–74 years	+3.9	−25.1 to +82.2	11	8	1	NS
75+ years	+9.2	−41.1 to +185.1	14	5	1	NS
Females[c]						
15–24 years	+6.0	−63.3 to +124.0	11	7	0	NS
25–34 years	+19.8	−25.0 to +77.8	14	4	0	$P = .03$
35–44 years	+15.4	−37.7 to +112.6	12	5	1	NS
45–54 years	+4.8	−23.8 to +94.9	11	7	0	NS
55–64 years	−9.3	−27.7 to +45.0	6	11	1	NS
65–74 years	+7.8	−20.7 to +46.2	13	5	0	NS
75+ years	+11.5	−28.7 to +67.5	12	6	0	NS

Note: [a] Sign test, two-tailed.
[b] Based on 20 countries (Iceland, Ireland, Luxembourg and Northern Ireland excluded).
[c] Based on 18 countries (Greece, Iceland, Ireland, Luxembourg, Norway and Northern Ireland excluded).
Source: (From Platt, 1989.)

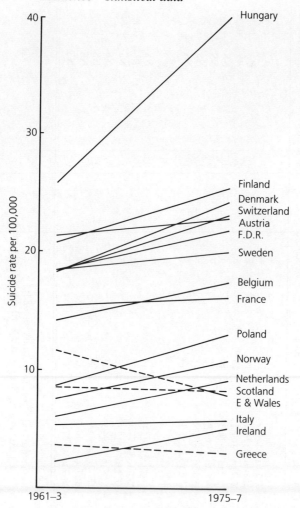

Figure 4.5. European suicide rates per 100,000: mean 1961–63 and mean 1975–77 (from Kreitman, 1980).

a corresponding trend has been expected in the European countries. Platt believes, on the basis of the figures that have been presented, that this development has not yet arrived. However, the development in Norway is clearly heading in this direction.

We must, however, pay close attention to the British situation. There has been a decline in the suicide trend in Great Britain if we look at the long-term development. A Figure from Kreitman (1980) (Figure 4.5) on the British anomaly is given here to illustrate this point.

This Figure shows that the suicide rate only fell in two countries in Europe over the period 1961–63 and 1975–77, and the clearest development was in Great Britain. Kreitman is of the opinion that the sharp decline there may be connected with the detoxification of domestic gas. This has traditionally been a very popular method of suicide in Great Britain, at one time accounting for 25% of all deaths from suicide. Domestic gas previously contained 14% carbon monoxide, but was purified or replaced by natural gas during the course of the 1960s, and by 1971 or 1972 the content of carbon monoxide was virtually zero. The gas consequently became far less dangerous from the point of view of suicide. The use of domestic gas as a way of committing suicide fell significantly in both sexes, as shown by Figure 4.6, and not least Figure 4.7, which shows the sharp decline which appears to have followed the period of detoxification. Lester (1990) shows that the detoxification of domestic gas in Switzerland was correlated with a decrease in the suicide rate as well as with a decrease in the use of domestic gas to commit suicide.

Corresponding data from the USA concerning the availability of firearms appear to show just as clearly that if the availability of firearms is reduced, the number of suicides from shooting and indeed the total sum of suicides is reduced. In the USA, firearms are used as a method of suicide in more than half of male suicides and in around a third of female suicides – far higher proportions than for example, in the Nordic

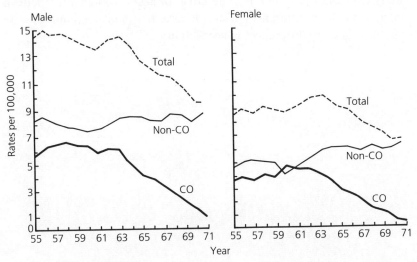

Figure 4.6. England and Wales: sex specific suicide rates by mode of death (from Kreitman, 1980).

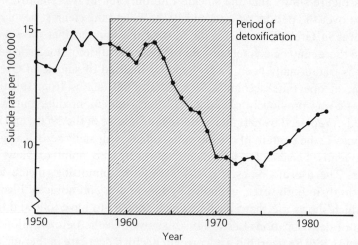

Figure 4.7. Male suicide rate (all ages) England and Wales: 1950–82

countries. Lester (1972) and Lester & Murel (1982), plus many others, have pointed out that the ready availability of firearms in the USA contributes to this, and that an important suicide prevention measure in the USA would be to be make the availability of firearms more difficult. Rich *et al*. (1990) and Sloan *et al*. (1990) found a reduction in suicide rates among the 15–24 age group when handguns were restricted. A recent study (Marzuk *et al*., 1992) of the effect of access to lethal methods of injury found that differences in suicide rates between communities were largely related to differences in accessibility.

5

Suicide in the Nordic countries

I shall concentrate on what the pattern of development has been like over a long period, and then assess in particular the trends over the last 25 years. It should be noted first of all that suicide is a major cause of death in the Nordic countries (i.e. Norway, Denmark, Finland, Sweden and Iceland, and including Greenland and Faroes). The latest available statistics show that 5003 suicides per year are registered in the Nordic region (1541 in Sweden, 1402 in Finland, 1378 in Denmark, 660 in Norway and 22 in Iceland; NOMESKO, 1991).

Suicide in the Nordic countries over a hundred-year period (1880–1980)

It can be seen from Figure 5.1 that Denmark has held a leading position virtually throughout this period, with a dip during the First World War, and sharing the position with Finland and Sweden during the last twenty years of this period.

In Figure 5.1 it can be seen that during the last century Finland had the lowest suicide rate, which then increased steadily, reaching the same level as Norway at the turn of the century and since around 1920 has shown a fairly sharp rise, with stagnation – or periods of decline – around the First and Second World Wars. In 1980 the figures were fairly equal for Denmark and Finland. Although Sweden until around 1920 had the second highest suicide rate among the Nordic countries, it was overtaken by Finland. Norway has come bottom since 1900, with the lowest values around the First World War and a steadily increasing rate since – an increase which has been more regular and constant than in the other

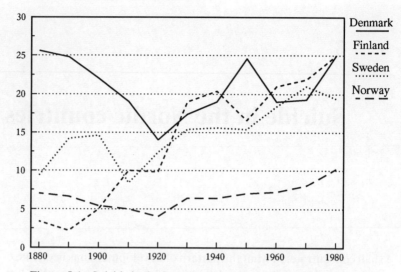

Figure 5.1. Suicide in the Scandinavian countries 1880–1980. Rates per 100,000.

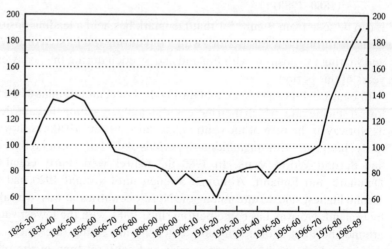

Figure 5.2. Suicide in Norway from 1826 to 1989 (from Gjertsen, 1987).

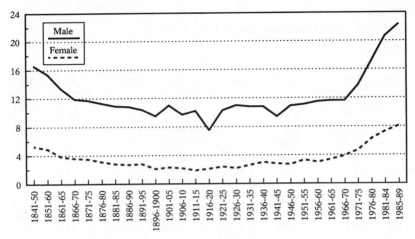

Figure 5.3. Suicide in Norway per 100,000 men and women in the period 1841–1989 (from Gjertsen, 1987).

Nordic countries. The trends in Norway are shown in Figures 5.2 and 5.3 and in Tables 5.1 to 5.4.

Where did the Scandinavian countries stand in the European context in the middle of the last century?

This is shown in Figure 5.4. It can be see that Sweden was at the lower end of the scale, after Iceland, whilst Norway was at the upper end, with Denmark occupying a special position as the leading suicide country in Europe, with a suicide rate more than twice as high as that of Norway and Prussia.

Development from 1966 to 1980

Let us now look at developments in more recent times. Since it appears that major changes occurred in the mid–1960s, we shall first focus on the period 1966–80. This is illustrated in Figure 5.5.

As can be seen from Figure 5.5, there was a steady increase in Denmark and Finland in this period from around 20 to 30 per 100,000, and in Norway from around eight to 12 per 100,000, whilst for Sweden there has been relatively little change. The latter may be partly explained by the fact that a decision was taken in Sweden in 1969 to classify all cases in which it was uncertain whether a death was suicidal or accidental in a

48   *Suicide in the Nordic countries*

Table 5.1. *Suicide rate per 100,000 of the indigenous population (1826–1985) in Norway*

Year	Rate	Year	Rate	Year	Rate	Year	Rate
		1865	8.5	1905	6.1	1945	9.2
1826	7.5	1866	7.1	1906	5.2	1946	6.1
1827	9.2	1867	7.6	1907	5.8	1947	6.5
1828	9.8	1868	7.5	1908	5.7	1948	6.9
1829	6.3	1869	7.6	1909	6.0	1949	6.6
1830	7.4	1870	8.5	1910	6.3	1950	7.4
1831	8.3	1871	7.3	1911	5.6	1951	6.5
1832	9.2	1872	7.5	1912	6.6	1952	6.9
1833	10.7	1873	7.1	1913	6.4	1953	7.6
1834	9.2	1874	7.8	1914	5.1	1954	7.4
1835	11.1	1875	8.0	1915	5.9	1955	7.4
1836	8.6	1876	7.8	1916	4.6	1956	7.3
1837	10.2	1877	7.0	1917	4.6	1957	7.4
1838	12.7	1878	7.0	1918	3.8	1958	7.3
1839	11.4	1879	7.4	1919	5.3	1959	7.9
1840	10.9	1880	6.5	1920	5.0	1960	6.5
1841	11.8	1881	6.4	1921	6.6	1961	6.6
1842	11.3	1882	7.1	1922	6.2	1962	7.9
1843	9.6	1883	6.9	1923	6.5	1963	8.0
1844	9.3	1884	6.7	1924	6.1	1964	7.3
1845	11.5	1885	6.6	1925	5.8	1965	7.7
1846	10.9	1886	6.7	1926	6.3	1966	7.1
1847	10.3	1887	6.7	1927	5.8	1967	7.0
1848	10.3	1888	7.1	1928	6.6	1968	8.1
1849	10.8	1889	6.6	1929	6.5	1969	8.2
1850	12.5	1890	6.3	1930	7.2	1970	8.4
1851	12.2	1891	6.0	1931	6.9	1971	8.1
1852	12.2	1892	6.4	1932	6.5	1972	9.0
1853	9.5	1893	6.4	1933	6.2	1973	8.7
1854	10.0	1894	7.1	1934	6.9	1974	10.4
1855	9.5	1895	6.6	1935	6.4	1975	9.9
1856	8.6	1896	5.7	1936	6.3	1976	10.8
1857	11.1	1897	4.8	1937	6.8	1977	11.4
1858	10.0	1898	6.4	1938	6.9	1978	11.7
1859	9.2	1899	6.0	1939	6.7	1979	12.1
1860	8.0	1900	5.5	1940	7.1	1980	12.4
1861	9.0	1901	6.2	1941	4.3	1981	12.8
1862	9.0	1902	6.6	1942	5.0	1982	14.0
1863	8.4	1903	6.7	1943	5.7	1983	14.6
1864	7.7	1904	6.9	1944	5.6	1984	14.5
						1985	14.1

Source: (From Gjertsen, 1987.)

Table 5.2. *Suicide and self-inflicted injury per 100,000 inhabitants in Norway*

	Total	Men	Women
1970	8.4	11.8	5.0
1971	8.1	12.3	4.0
1972	9.0	13.0	5.1
1973	8.7	13.1	4.3
1974	10.4	16.3	4.5
1975	9.9	14.2	5.6
1976	10.8	16.0	5.6
1977	11.4	16.9	5.9
1978	11.7	17.4	6.0
1979	12.1	17.2	7.1
1980	12.4	18.3	6.7
1981	12.8	19.1	6.5
1982	14.0	20.7	7.5
1983	14.6	21.2	8.1
1984	14.5	21.9	7.2
1985	14.1	20.8	7.4
1986	13.9	20.3	7.6
1987	15.5	23.5	7.7

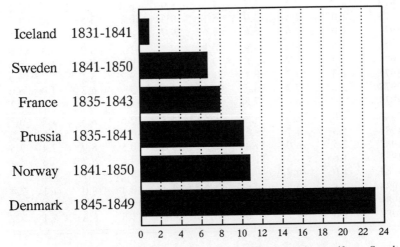

Figure 5.4. Registered suicides per 100,000 inhabitants (from Sundt, 1855).

Table 5.3. *Frequency of suicide per 100,000 by sex and age in Norway from 1970 to 1987*

Sex Year	Age group 10–19	20–29	30–39	40–49	50–59	60–69	70–79	80+	Total
Men									
1970	1.0	10.9	17.1	16.6	23.8	21.3	17.5	17.6	11.8
1971	1.6	11.6	12.2	26.9	20.2	21.0	17.2	17.4	12.3
1972	3.8	12.0	15.0	23.2	20.9	23.5	20.6	17.1	13.0
1973	5.1	9.5	18.3	21.6	26.6	18.3	14.8	30.6	13.1
1974	4.1	18.0	19.8	24.1	32.8	28.6	16.4	16.2	16.3
1975	5.0	17.0	13.3	24.2	24.1	18.8	27.9	15.8	14.2
1976	7.2	15.1	15.8	26.7	28.8	24.3	25.0	25.5	16.0
1977	7.4	18.7	21.0	26.1	28.2	21.5	23.8	32.2	16.9
1978	4.9	22.0	23.4	24.8	28.2	25.8	21.7	21.7	17.4
1979	4.6	24.9	15.8	22.4	34.6	27.6	18.8	18.7	17.2
1980	8.1	22.6	19.8	24.3	30.5	26.9	25.1	27.5	18.3
1981	6.0	24.4	24.5	26.7	34.4	24.6	24.7	15.7	19.1
1982	9.2	24.0	22.6	32.8	25.7	30.3	21.0	26.4	20.7
1983	9.8	26.8	19.3	28.1	43.8	29.2	25.4	23.6	21.2
1984	8.6	28.5	23.5	29.2	33.3	38.8	25.7	16.8	21.9
1985	9.3	28.6	27.8	26.4	33.6	21.4	26.2	20.7	20.8
1986	10.1	25.2	26.5	28.2	30.2	24.8	22.1	22.5	20.3
1987	8.1	32.2	24.5	32.1	32.8	33.9	29.4	44.1	23.5
Women									
1970	0.7	4.4	5.0	11.4	9.6	7.9	4.5	1.9	5.0
1971	1.0	5.3	6.1	6.5	6.1	5.9	4.4	1.9	4.0
1972	0.7	8.3	5.5	7.6	8.9	6.8	7.8	–	5.1
1973	1.0	4.4	3.9	5.1	9.3	10.4	3.5	–	4.3
1974	1.0	4.0	5.6	7.6	9.7	8.5	2.7	3.4	4.5
1975	1.0	6.4	5.8	10.2	8.5	11.2	6.0	3.3	5.6
1976	1.3	7.7	3.8	9.4	13.5	9.3	3.3	1.6	5.6
1977	1.3	7.7	8.1	11.1	9.5	9.2	5.1	–	5.9
1978	2.3	7.7	8.5	8.1	13.0	5.9	6.3	1.4	6.0
1979	0.6	8.4	7.5	14.7	14.9	11.7	5.0	1.4	7.1
1980	1.0	8.4	5.8	8.6	14.3	12.5	8.5	1.3	6.7
1981	1.3	4.7	8.5	9.6	16.5	10.5	6.6	2.5	6.5
1982	2.5	6.0	11.4	12.5	13.8	10.5	8.9	2.4	7.5
1983	1.6	4.3	11.1	14.7	16.0	14.8	8.7	5.8	8.1
1984	1.6	6.9	6.7	11.8	13.6	13.9	8.1	6.7	7.2
1985	2.5	10.7	8.6	11.2	12.4	10.4	8.0	1.1	7.4
1986	1.6	3.5	10.6	12.3	16.2	12.6	11.2	2.1	7.6
1987	1.6	7.7	7.6	14.5	14.9	11.5	8.3	5.1	7.7

Table 5.4. *Cause of death according sex for the age group 14–24 in Norway, 1987*

(ICD-9) Cause of death		15–24 years	%
Total number of deaths	M	357	100
	W	111	100
Total number of deaths by disease	M	79	22
	W	52	47
Cardio-vascular disease (390–459)	M	31	9
	W	9	8
Cancers (150–208)	M	26	7
	W	15	14
Other diseases	M	22	6
	W	28	25
Total number of deaths by violence	M	278	78
	W	59	53
Traffic accidents involving motor vehicles (E810–E819)	M	119	33
	W	30	27
Suicide (E950–E959)	M	80	22
	W	12	11
Other violent deaths	M	79	22
	W	17	15

Note: ICD-9 = International classification of diseases, 9th revision (WHO, 1977).
M = men   W = women
(*Source:* Central Bureau of Statistics of Norway, 1987.)

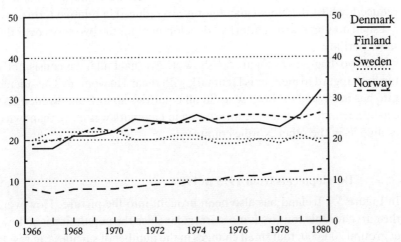

Figure 5.5. Suicide in the Scandinavian countries 1966–80. Rates per 100,000.

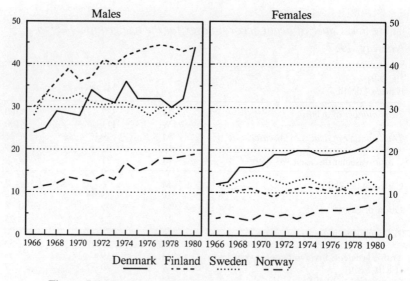

Figure 5.6. Suicide in the Scandinavian countries 1966–80, according to sex. Rates per 100,000.

special group, and not under suicide, as had been the case previously. This group has since been considerably larger in Sweden than in the other countries, and accounts for around a third of cases of suicide (seven to eight per 100,000), whilst it represents only one per 100,000 in Norway and three to four per 100,000 in Denmark and Finland. If this group is included, the difference between Sweden and Denmark–Finland is reduced, whilst the Norwegian figures are reduced in relative terms.

I shall now assess the pattern of development for the two sexes over the same period.

The two diagrams of Figure 5.6 show clearly that Finland is consistently top with regard to men, as is Denmark with regard to women. The suicide rate has increased for both sexes in all countries apart from Sweden. As can be seen, the suicide rate for women in Denmark was more than twice as high as in the other Nordic countries.

Developments from 1975 to 1989

In Figure 5.7 Iceland has also been brought into the picture. However, the curve for this country is more irregular since the population is so low, at around 200,000, that small changes in the number of suicides can result in wide fluctuations in the statistics. It can be seen that Denmark and

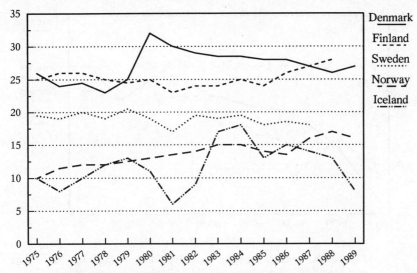

Figure 5.7. Suicides in the Nordic countries 1975–89, per 100,000 inhabitants (Sweden to 1987; Finland to 1988).
Sources: NOMESKO. Health Statistics for the Nordic countries (several volumes); T. Gjertsen. Suicide in Norway. 1987: 103; Danish Health statistics (T. Barfoed personal info.); High scool of Iceland (G. Baldursson personal info.); Central Bureau of Statistics (Y. Lönn personal info.); Statistikcentralen (H. Ahonen personal info.).

Finland stay close together at the top, whilst an increase also takes place in Norway, fairly evenly throughout the period, and Iceland more or less follows the trend in Norway. Sweden is also in mid-table during this period (around 20), with a slight change from year to year.

Development trends in relation to age and sex 1988

I shall now analyse the age distribution, first among men.

Figure 5.8 shows that the numbers have risen for the 20–29 age group and that the Norwegian figures for the youngest age groups (up to 29 years) are just as high as or even higher than those of Denmark and Sweden, with only Finland clearly higher.

However, the Finnish figures show a drop for the 80+ age group, where a clear increase is apparent for Norway, Sweden and Denmark, and in the group aged over 70 the Danish figures are clearly the highest.

The pattern of development among women is different, as Figure 5.9 shows. There is a fairly similar pattern between the countries up to the

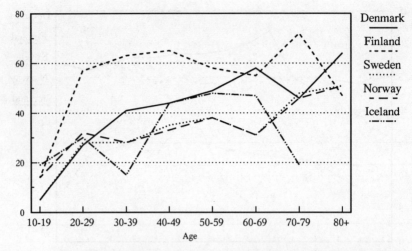

Figure 5.8. Suicides among men according to age in the Nordic countries 1988. Age groups per 100,000 inhabitants (Sweden 1987). *Sources:* SBB.NOS. Cause of death 1988; Danish Health statistics (T. Barfoed personal info.); High scool of Iceland (G. Baldursson personal info.); Central Bureau of Statistics (Y. Lönn personal info.); Statistikcentralen (H. Ahonen personal info.).

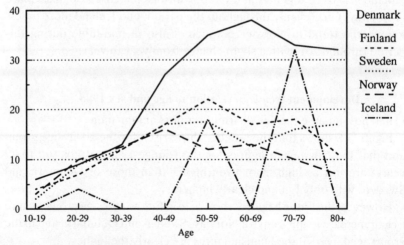

Figure 5.9. Suicides among women according to age in the Nordic countries 1988. Age groups per 100,000 inhabitants (Sweden 1987). *Sources:* see Fig. 5.8.

30–39 age group, but thereafter the curve rises steeply for Denmark, which has a clear lead in all upper age groups, followed by Finland. There is a slight falling trend for all countries from the 50–60 age group, but with a slight trend towards an increase in Sweden. There are thus clear differences for the two sexes between the countries.

Development of suicide for the youngest age groups (age 15–24) in the period 1966–80.

Figure 5.10 shows that the suicide rate in Sweden for the period studied has fluctuated little whereas Norway, Sweden and Finland have marked increases, with Norway having relatively the greatest increase. Finland has remained consistently higher than any of the other three countries.

The pattern of development by sex is shown in Figure 5.11. It can be seen here that Finland has easily the highest suicide rate in this age group among men, with a peak in the 1970s, but has also had high figures since then. It can also be seen that the increase was greatest in Norway, which overtook Sweden and Denmark in 1980. With regard to women, Denmark does not hold the leading position in this age group, as would be expected from its leading position in suicide among women. It is women aged over 30 who account for Denmark's leading position.

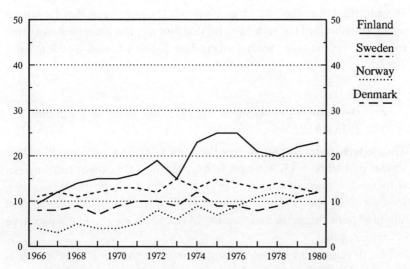

Figure 5.10. Suicide in the Scandinavian countries 1966–80. 15 to 24-year-olds. Rates per 100,000.

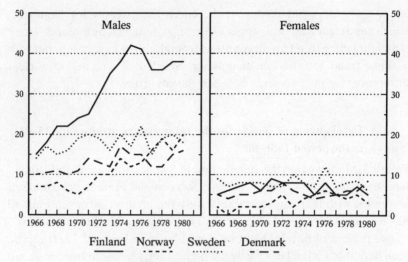

Figure 5.11. Suicide in the Scandinavian countries 1966–80. 15 to 24-year-olds, according to sex. Rates per 100,000.

Development of suicide in the youngest age group (15–19) over the period 1975–89

Figure 5.12 shows the pattern of development for the very youngest (15–19 year olds) over the last 15 year period. It can be seen that Finland is again well ahead of the rest, but also that Norway has witnessed easily the most steady increase, having overtaken Denmark and Sweden since 1987.

Development of suicide in the 15–29 age group in the period 1975–89

The pattern of development over the same period for men aged 15–29 is shown in Figure 5.13. Finland is in a league of its own, but has not witnessed a marked increase over the period. A particularly sharp increase over the period is shown by Norway, which has moved well ahead of both Denmark and Sweden. As can be seen, the Icelandic curve is very irregular.

The development among young women in the 15–29 age group is shown in Figure 5.14. It can be seen here that Denmark holds a leading position over a major part of the period, closely followed by Sweden and

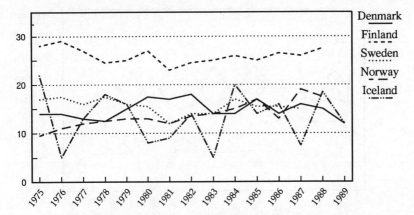

Figure 5.12. Suicide in 15–19 age group in the Nordic countries 1975–89. Rates per 100,000 inhabitants (Sweden to 1987; Finland to 1988).
Sources: see Fig. 5.8.

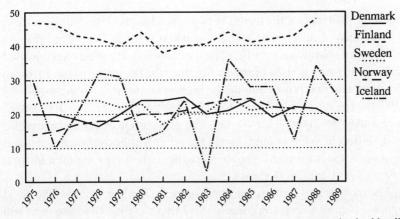

Figure 5.13. Suicide among men in the 15–29 age group in the Nordic countries 1975–89. Rates per 100,000 inhabitants (Sweden to 1987; Finland to 1988).
Sources: see Fig. 5.8.

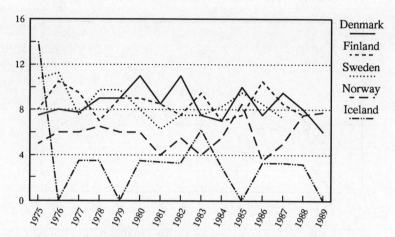

Figure 5.14. Suicide among women in the 15–29 age group in the Nordic countries 1975–89. Rates per 100,000 inhabitants (Sweden to 1987; Finland to 1988).
Sources: see Fig. 5.8.

Finland, and in the last few years of the period also by Norway. The Icelandic figures are too 'untidy' to be commented on.

Two special areas in the Nordic region: Greenland and the Faeroes

Finally I shall look at the trends in two special parts of the Nordic region. The pattern of development that has taken place in Greenland (Figure 5.15) sets it apart from the other Nordic countries. It can be seen how that the suicide rate has risen dramatically since the beginning of the 1970s, to the point where it is now among the highest known rates in the world. By 1987 the suicide rate had risen to 127. The figure was 173 per 100,000 for men and 64 per 100,000 for women. The distribution by sex and age is also quite different in Greenland than in the other Nordic countries. Suicide is to a great extent a youth problem, particularly for young men in their twenties, as Figure 5.16 shows.

The trend is also shown clearly in Figure 5.17, which includes the latest figures. It can be seen from Figure 5.17 that the ratio between men and women is around 3:1, as in Norway. Suicide accounts for around 19% of all deaths in men and 10% in women, and is a very common cause of death in Greenland, more common than in any other Nordic country. As

Period	Annual average	Annual average per 100,000 inhabitans
1891-1930	0.4	4
1951-1960	3.0	11
1962-1966	7.0	19
1967-1971	6.0	17
1972-1976	22.0	54
1977-1981	32.0	74
1982-1986	52.0	117

Up to 1964 the registered number of suicides represents the whole population. Thereafter the Greenland-born population only.

Figure 5.15. Number of suicides registered in Greenland in the period 1890–1986.
Sources: Grove & Lynge, 1979; Lynge, 1982; Bertelsen, 1935; Social Kritik, 1989.

can also be seen, suicide, murder and accidents, that is violent deaths, account for more than a third of all deaths among men and almost a fifth of all deaths among women.

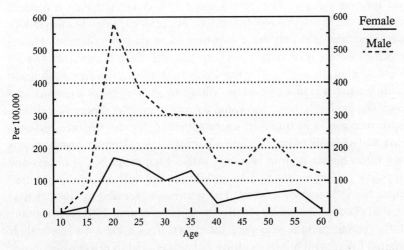

Figure 5.16. Ages and suicide in Greenland. Average per year 1977–86.
Source: Social Kritik, No. 4, 1989.

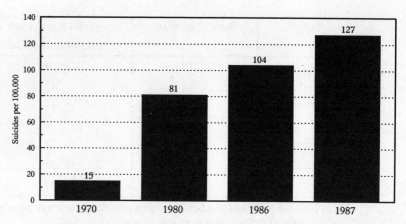

In 1987: 178 for men, 64 for women.

Suicides represent at least 18.9% of all deaths of men, 9.8% of women.
Overall, suicides, homicides and accidents cause 37.7% of all deaths
of men, 16.5% of women.

Figure 5.17. Frequency of suicides in Greenland, per 100,000.
Source: Årbog for Grønland, 1988 (Ministry of State, The Greenland
Dept).

It is logical to conclude that the sharp rise and high rate is due to culture
clashes. Greenland has undergone profound social changes since colonial
status was abolished in 1953. From a protected existence with a fishing
and hunting culture, Greenland was to be converted into a modern
society in the shortest possible time. Considerable trained Danish labour
was imported, and may have contributed to the Greenlanders feeling
inferior in their own country. There has also been a concentration of
population in the towns. The transition from a poor but free fishing and
hunting existence in a Greenland village to a tower-block existence in a
town has probably been too rapid for many people. There has been a
sharp increase in alcoholism, unemployment, the use of force, promiscuity and a feeling of hopelessness. Per capita the alcohol consumption is
four times higher than in Norway, with a high incidence of binges and
excessive drunkenness. Nearly all killings and suicides are committed
under the influence of alcohol. The impression formed by doctors who
have worked in Greenland (N. Bratberg, pers. comm. 1991) is that many
of the young people who take their own lives appear to reject their
original fishing and hunting culture but also appear to reject tower-block
and factory life in the new western culture which is becoming established
there.

The figures from the Faeroes – the 'low-incidence area' in the Nordic region (Wang, 1989) – are in sharp contrast to those from Greenland. The incidence of suicide on the Faeroes was around three per 100,000 until 1970, but has increased to between six and seven over the last few years, well below half that in Norway. The ratio between men and women is 3:1, as in Norway. The Faeroes are the part of the Nordic region that has retained its traditions and values the best, isolated as the country is far out in the Atlantic Ocean.

Some concluding remarks

Let me conclude this presentation of statistics with a few words about the ratio between men and women. This is also striking and interesting in the Nordic region. The ratio in Finland is 4:1. This was also the ratio in Norway a hundred years ago, but the ratio there is now 3:1, and has remained fairly steady at this level from year to year in all age groups, apart from the very old (over 80), where the ratio is 6:1. In Sweden, the ratio has fallen from 3:1 to 2.4:1, but the ratio in Denmark is 1.7:1. The ratio in Denmark has always shown a relatively high incidence among women in comparison with the other Nordic countries.

What about the geographical differences? In this brief survey I cannot discuss how the situation has developed in the various geographical areas. Differences between town and country and between the various parts of the country exist in all the Nordic countries. Just as in Europe the greatest increase in suicide is found in countries which have traditionally been low-incidence countries, the same trend has been detected in Norway – a sharper increase in the low-incidence country of Norway in comparison with the high-incidence countries of Denmark and Finland. The same trend is apparent within each country. It is in the villages, which traditionally have had low suicide rates, that the increase is now sharpest, and it is highest in relative terms in the villages and also counties where the suicide rates have been low. In Norway this has been clearly detected among young people. Over a seven-year period (1975–81), the suicide statistics were thoroughly analysed for young people in Oslo aged 15–29 (Retterstøl, Ekeland & Hessø, 1985). The absolute figure was 148. An increase was expected here. The figures for the next seven-year period (1982–88) are now available – 142, that is a fall rather than a rise. There has been a three-fold increase in this age group on a national basis. This increase has not come from Oslo or from the few other large towns in Norway. If the Norwegian figures are analysed more closely in these age groups, we find that the four largest towns (Oslo, Bergen, Trondheim and Stavanger) show no or only a moderate increase, lower than the rest of the country. The increase has been greatest in the three northern counties, with a dramatic doubling of the rate in Finnmark (see Jørgensen, 1991).

There are thus vast differences in the problem of suicide in the Nordic countries. By European standards they are 'high-incidence countries', with Finland and Denmark at the top, well up in the 20s for registered suicides per 100,000 inhabitants with Finland close to being the top country for men and Denmark for women. Sweden comes well behind with just under 20, and Norway and Iceland with around 15 – with the sharpest and most consistent rise in Norway, which can be expected to reach the general Nordic level. However, this small part of the world also includes Greenland with 127 and the Faeroes with just under seven. It is not surprising that the Nordic countries themselves and the rest of the world continue to be obsessed with the problems of suicide in the Nordic region.

The WHO has defined its long-term targets in the programme 'Health for all by the year 2000'. Target 12 states: 'By the year 2000 the incidence of suicide and attempted suicide must be turned round from the current increase to a reduction' (Helsedirektoratet, 1987). The target is clear and positive. But there are only eight years to go. There are major tasks ahead in the Nordic countries.

Suicidal attempts in the Nordic countries

The term attempted suicide, as used throughout this book, includes also what has been previously referred to as parasuicide (see chapter 1). During the 1960s and 1970s attempted suicide clearly emerges as a major challenge facing the health services in most countries of the western world (Kreitman, 1977; Hawton & Catalan, 1987).

There is no central registration of attempted suicides in the Nordic countries, a situation which is similar in other European countries. A WHO (Euro) Multicenter Study on Parasuicide is now being performed in 16 centres in Europe. Preliminary findings from this study have been presented by Platt (1990). In 1989 the event rates (i.e. rates of suicidal attempts) for males varied from 414 per 100,000 in Helsinki (Finland) to 47 in Leiden (the Netherlands). Sør-Trøndelag in Norway was in the middle, 169 per 100,000, that is about ten times higher than the suicide incidence for Norway.

The highest female event rate was 595 in Pontoise (France) and the lowest 95 in Guipuzcoa (Spain). The female:male ratio varied from 0.71:1 to 2.15:1, with a median of 1.46:1 (events). The female:male ratio in Sør-Trøndelag was 1.34. In addition, some preliminary findings have been reported from single centres (Ostamo & Lønnquist, 1990; Prins & Kerkhof, 1990; Crepet *et al.*, 1990; Querejeta *et al.*, 1990; De Leo, 1990). As in other centres in Europe, Bjerke, Rygnestad & Stiles (1991) found the rates higher among 20 to 29-year-olds. The rates in Sør-Trøndelag was lowest among those over 60 years of age. This later finding was consistent with the results from most other European centres (Platt, 1990), but some centres (Crepet *et al.*, 1990; Querejeta, 1990) report higher rates for those over 65 years of age. Bjerke *et al.* (1991) found that in Norway patients who had attempted suicide had a considerable higher migrating activity than the general population. They were also more often than expected divorced or separated, and less often married. They had a relatively low level of education and a high proportion of the males were unemployed, while females were more often economically inactive.

The results of the Norwegian study of non-fatal repetion of attempted suicide were to a large extent consistent with earlier research (Kreitman, 1988). Male attempted suicide patients were characterized by having more social, economic, criminal and alcohol and drug dependency problems than female attempted suicide patients. Rygnestad (1990) has shown that the rate of self-poisoning at the Regional Hospital of Trondheim increased gradually over the period from 1940 to 1987. He compared patients admitted after deliberate self-poisoning in 1978 with patients admitted in 1987, and found that family problems, unemployment, poor social conditions and alcohol and drug abuse had increased in importance during this period.

Interesting results have been reported from Finland (Ostamo & Lønnquist, 1991) where the WHO study was started in four different, clearly defined catchment areas. All attempted suicides admitted to the health care system in these areas were systematically registered over one year. The male/female ratio of absolute numbers in all areas was about 1:1, very different from the results in other countries. The age profile was similar in the four areas – most cases in the age group 25–39 years. Almost half of the patients were unmarried. The results tentatively showed that there were local variations to the attempted suicide rate as for the suicide rate, and was more than ten times higher than the rate for successful suicides.

High attempted suicide rates in cities and big towns give the suggestion that there are some factors provoking the attempted suicide behaviour in addition to the classical social causes. These could be a self-destructive life-style, better possibilities to communicate by using suicidal behaviour and many human contacts to learn attempted suicide behaviour as coping behaviour.

Suicide attempts within specific areas in Sweden have been described by Salander-Renberg & Jacobsson (1991) for Västerbotten county and for the Stockholm area by Wasserman & Eklund (1991). In the later study the attempted suicide rate was 260 (205 were male and 310 were female). The peak for attempted suicide rates was in the slightly older age groups than previous investigations have shown (25–34 age group in female, 45–54 age group in male). In Stockholm there was found an exceptionally high attempted suicide rate among Finnish citizens (513) resident there, especially in the 15–34 year age group (726). This is reported for the first time in Sweden. In both studies it was demonstrated that divorced and widowed people had very high attempted suicide rates.

In *Suicide Attempts in the Nordic Countries* (ed. Bjerke & Stiles, 1991) treatment procedures are also discussed, as are preventive measures. The national programme for suicide prevention in Norway has now been presented (Ekeberg, 1992).

6

Why is the suicide rate lower in Norway than in the other Nordic countries?

This question has interested the world, precisely because the Nordic countries are so similar. I shall first look at some earlier international studies which have been regarded as essential to this discussion, namely the books written by Hendin and Farber (Hendin, 1967; Farber, 1968). I shall also discuss sociological and demographic theories, and finally examine the results of a six-year research project conducted under the auspices of the Nordic Planning Group for Suicide Research, set up by the Nordic Co-operative Board for Medical Research (NOS-M).

Hendin's theory

The book *Suicide and Scandinavia* by American psychiatrist H. Hendin dating from 1964 has aroused considerable international attention. His book is based on a relatively short stay in Denmark, Norway and Sweden (around six months in each of the countries) and in the capitals. He interviewed a limited number of patients with suicide problems – around 25 people from each country who had attempted suicide. In addition he interviewed psychiatric patients who had not attempted suicide and also nurses in hospitals. He also tried to obtain broad information on the literature and history in these countries. He puts forward the view that there are different patterns of suicide in the three countries, and a different background to these patterns. In particular he interpreted the differences on the basis of *different patterns in the upbringing of children and the triggering of aggression in the three countries*.

He believes that the suicides in Sweden are marked by the Swedish personality traits of rigidity, a high level of ambition, severe anxiety and a feeling of guilt about not being adequate. These features, he believes, are in turn related to early mother–child separation. Swedish mothers according to Hendin are ambitious, obsessed with their own self-realisation and progress and do not have time or cannot afford to be at home to give the child sufficient love and affection in their formative years. The prototype of a suicide in Sweden is what he calls *the performance type of suicide*.

In Denmark, according to his theory, suicide is primarily related to a 'loss of dependency'. He is of the opinion that the child in Denmark is made too dependent on its mother, who will herself be the centre-point and bind the child to herself. The personality pattern in Denmark is said to be characterised by the fact that people suppress their aggression and engender a feeling of guilt in others, but do not display their aggression outwardly. It is a form of 'smiling' aggression. He calls the prototype of suicide in Denmark *dependency loss type of suicide*.

In contrast to these patterns, the upbringing of children in Norway is said to contribute to greater independence and a greater ability to come forward with aggression and other feelings openly. He believes that Norwegians are better able to express aggression than Danes and Swedes. He also believed that he found a specific Norwegian type of suicide which he called the *moral* form of suicide, which stemmed from aggressive, antisocial behaviour, accompanied by strong feelings of guilt as a result of the puritanical and pietistic attitudes held in many places in Norway.

A great deal of criticism can be levelled at Hendin's work. Firstly, he accepted the Scandinavian suicide statistics at face value and did not subject them to critical examination. Secondly, it is not suicide that he is concerned with in his survey but those who attempt suicide who, many people believe, differ from those who commit suicide. Thirdly, it is a highly dubious practice to analyse the national character in countries. The objection can be made that there may be just as wide differences in the character of the people and methods of bringing up children between districts within the same country as between related nations. His observations can, however, be regarded as interesting reflections.

Farber's theory

Farber, an American, was of the view that there are differences in the pattern of bringing up children between Denmark and Norway, as he described in his book *Theory of Suicide* (1968). He only studied the differences between Denmark and Norway. He holds the view that the Norwegian mother is very preoccupied with giving her child a correct upbringing and giving it love and affection, and also believes that the Norwegian father is stricter and holds a more central position in the family than his Danish counterpart. He comes to the conclusion that warmth and affection in the primary group – the family – is greater in Norway than in Denmark, and believes that this is a major factor in the incidence of suicide being so low in Norway. As I shall discuss later, some support has been found for this theory, which was not based on empirical research.

Sociological and demographic theories

The Finnish professor of sociology Erik Allardt from Helsinki made an interesting study of a number of variable data in the population of the four Nordic countries (Allardt, 1975). The data he recorded, and which are based on a fairly wide-ranging programme of research, are such phenomena as contentment, degree of cohesion with the group, the family, the nation, etc. His analyses in many ways fit in well with the Norwegian statistics referred to on the incidence of suicide. He found for example that the degree of satisfaction was greatest in Norway, as was the cohesion in the individual group, particularly family solidarity. He similarly found that a national sense of belonging, a feeling of identity with the nation, was significantly greater in Norway than in the other countries, the welfare society had advanced furthest in Sweden, and the degree of dissatisfaction was greatest in Finland. However, it was also high in Sweden. The most privatised society was that in Denmark. Here the sense of belonging in families was weakest and identity with the nation weakest. Allardt's work revealed clear sociological differences between the four Nordic countries, and gave possible clues to explaining the low incidence of suicide in Norway in comparison with the other countries.

There are also other studies which appear to show that Norway comes out favourably on a number of sociological factors. The Austrian study group for international analyses has examined a large quantity of data from a number of European countries (Fuchs, Gaspari & Millendorfer, 1977). The data relates to age at marriage, birth rate, divorce rate, sense of belonging in families and a number of social data concerned with family life. The Austrian family research group established quite clear correlations between the incidence of suicide in a country and sociological data relating to family life. On the basis of these indicators, the group produced the finding that there are two countries in western Europe which differ sharply with respect to a number of favourable factors: the Netherlands and Norway. Both these countries have a noticeably low incidence of suicide. The Austrian group believes that the reason for Norway's favourable position in the suicide statistics is that it has better and closer family relationships.

The latest study has been made by the American social anthropologist Raoul Narroll of Buffalo University, New York, in his book *The Moral Order* (Narroll, 1983). In this book he presents a model which is designed to assess what he termed moral norms in a society. He found that close family groups and smaller communities offered the best protection against different forms of socially deviant behaviour, such as suicide. He tried among a number of countries, with what is referred to as a high quality of life, to find a model country which was characterized by the norms which he believed to be most favourable for the prevention of undesirable behaviour. He used a large quantity of international statistics to identify this country. It was Norway that according to his methods, stood out as the 'model country' to follow. The 12 nations which he took for comparison were Canada, Denmark, Finland, West Germany, Iceland, Israel, Luxembourg, the Netherlands, Norway, Spain, Sweden and the USA. He based his analysis for all nations on official statistics from the United Nations or the WHO. He took 12 major areas of risk (parameters) to compare the countries (divorce rate, criminality, abuse of alcohol and drugs, etc.). Norway came out best on all 12 parameters, followed by Sweden and the Netherlands. His conclusion, based on the statistics, is as follows: 'In this way, I have chosen Norway as my model country. Furthermore, Norway not only is the nation with reportedly the best overall average on my twelve parameters; of the four leading nations on my list it is also the best balanced. The variance of its standard scores among the twelve parameters is the least. In other words Norway not only does best on the average overall, but it comes the nearest to doing fairly well on every individual parameter – avoiding extremes.'

I know from our Scandinavian statistics that Norway compares favourably with its Scandinavian neighbours in a number of areas, which to some extent also relate to the suicide rate. The divorce rate is substantially lower in Norway than in the other Nordic countries. Alcohol consumption per inhabitant is easily lowest in Norway. Criminality is lower, as is violent crime and the number of murders. Drug abuse among the young has not been as widespread in Norway as in Sweden and Denmark, whilst Finland probably has the same or a lower level.

Research results from the Nordic Planning Group for Suicide Research

Prompted by the fact that the suicide rate was rising in most European countries and was high in the Nordic countries, the Nordic Co-operative Board for Medical Research (NOS-M) decided in 1977 to set up a joint Nordic planning group on suicide research. The group comprised two researchers from each country, appointed by the national medical research councils. The author of this book was the chairman of the group for its first three years and Professor Juel-Nielsen from Denmark for the next three-year period. The group's work was completed in 1983 (Juel-Nielsen, Retterstøl & Bille-Brahe, 1987).

The Nordic research project had two main phases. The first phase of the project comprised a collection of statistical material and analyses of recording practice, principles and routines in both the reporting and recording systems in the individual Nordic countries. Practice was studied particularly with respect to whether the strikingly low incidence of suicide for recorded suicides in Norway might be due to differences in recording practice and statistical documentation between Norway and the other countries, or whether there was a real difference in the incidence of suicide.

The study contained detailed analyses of the forms of death and causes of death which could be assumed to 'conceal' cases of suicide. There are two types of potential sources of error. The first of these comprises drowning accidents. Drowning accidents occur more commonly in Norway and Finland than in the other Nordic countries. Skullberg (1974) made a detailed analysis of drowning accidents in Norway. He found that among 469 deaths due to drowning, 79 were registered as suicide. In a detailed examination of all cases of drowning accidents, he was able to find three cases of 'concealed' suicide, which must be considered to be a small number when it is borne in mind that the age composition was the same as the age composition for drowning accidents in other countries. There is always a large proportion of children among those who drown, and the ratio was the same in Norway as in the other countries.

The other source of error in the registration of suicide consisted of cases of doubt between suicide and accidents, and deaths where the cause of death is stated as being unknown. It was found, however, that the incidence of cases of doubt between suicide and accidents was highest in Sweden for both sexes and in all age groups and lowest in Norway. Even if the cases of doubt between accidents and suicide and the registered cases of suicide were combined, there was no major change in the overall rates in the Nordic countries. Another source of error in registration was made up of deaths which it was difficult to categorise in the cause of death statistics because of the lack of information on the background to the death. These are deaths registered as 'death from unknown cause' and as 'natural death of unknown cause'. Deaths which occurred suddenly and unexpectedly were common in both Norway and Denmark in all age groups, but most common in the oldest age groups. There were no grounds for suspecting that these deaths might be concealed suicides.

To summarise, the study of the reliability of the registration of suicide in the Nordic countries showed that registration is equally reliable in all four countries as far as the younger age groups below the age of 40 are concerned. Reliability was less certain for the older age groups, since there are potential sources of error. However, these sources of error were just as great in Denmark as in Norway, and the following conclusions have therefore been drawn.

Conclusions on the first phase of the project: The potential sources of error which exist are not of a sufficient order of magnitude to explain the differences in the registered suicide rates. In other words, there are significant differences between the rate of suicide in Norway and the rate of suicide in the other Nordic countries.

The second phase of the project: Aimed at identifying demographic, epidemiological, socio-cultural, psychological and other data which could be assumed to influence the suicide rate and variations in it. The Danish sociologist Unni Bille-Brahe prepared a model as an element in this phase of the research project (1987). An attempt was made in the project to assess the degree of social integration on the basis of data from the Nordic welfare studies. A model was constructed which could be used for a comparison of the level of social integration in the Nordic countries. A distinction was made in the assessment of the degree of social integration between the following main areas of life:

(1) Immediate environment
(2) Working life
(3) Social life in general

An integration index was prepared for each of the three areas, and the total social integration was measured by linking together the three indicators. For practical reasons a comparison was only made between Norway and Denmark.

A study was also made of whether the differences in the age and sex-specific suicide rate between Norway and Denmark can be explained on the basis of corresponding differences in the degree of social integration.

The results of the study have shown that the level of social integration is considerably lower in Denmark for both sexes, but particularly for women. The high level of integration in Norway is partly due to Norwegians having closer relationships with family and friends than the Danes and partly to their being more committed to their society, particularly at local level. The degree of social integration was found to be low in the groups characterised by a high suicide rate. Danish middle-aged women (i.e. age group 50–65) for example, are particularly poorly socially integrated, both in comparison with Danish women generally and particularly in comparison with Norwegian women in the same age group. Among young Norwegian men in the age group 20–9, who show a sharply rising suicide rate, the degree of integration declined over the period 1973–80.

The model was thus shown to be a suitable method for studying and comparing social integration. The model has given valuable experience which it will be possible to use as a basis for corresponding studies in the other Nordic countries.

The Nordic Planning Group for Suicide Research can therefore be said to have brought about a major advance in the comparison of suicide rates between the Nordic countries. The differences thus appear to be real, and there also appear to be sociological and cultural ways of explaining the differences. However, there are dark clouds on the horizon for Norwegians. The Norwegian suicide rate has risen regularly and steadily, and the sharpest rise in the incidence of suicide is among the young. It will therefore be no surprise if the suicide rate in Norway becomes just as high as in the other Scandinavian countries over the next ten years.

With regard to the reliability of suicide statistics in Norway, another study was published in 1975 which suggests that the Norwegian suicide statistics are quite reliable.

This study is by Ø. Ekeberg, F. Jacobsen and E. Enger, of Dept. VII, Ullevål Hospital, Oslo, P. Frederichsen of the Central Laboratory, Ullevål Hospital and L. Holand of the Norwegian Central Bureau of Statistics (Ekeberg, Frederichsen & Holan, 1985). An internal medicine specialist, a psychiatrist and a toxicologist each independently examined

210 forensic autopsy records to assess whether any were cases of *definite* suicide, *possible* suicide or *unlikely* suicide. The assessments were compared with the official death certificates as registered by the Central Bureau of Statistics. The intention was to obtain an impression of the extent to which there is under-registration in the two main groups of sudden death covered by the study, deaths from poisoning and drowning, which account for some 40% of suicides in Norway. This possibility has been put forward to explain the low suicide figures in Norway compared with its neighbours, as discussed earlier. On the basis of the number of definite suicides in the retrospective assessment, the study did not provide any evidence of official under-registration. If cases where there could be doubt were also included, there was an official under-registration of around 10% for the selected material. This is such a low figure that it will not have any significant effect on Norwegian suicide statistics. The study therefore provides little reason to assume that the official Norwegian suicide statistics reflect any under-reporting. It is assumed that in the total statistics for all methods of suicide, the percentage of under-registration will be lower than 10%.

The study therefore supports the official suicide statistics, which show that the incidence of suicide is significantly lower in Norway than in Denmark, Finland and Sweden.

The results obtained by the Nordic research group have been published in supplement no. 336 to *Acta Psychiatrica Scandinavica* (Juel-Nielsen *et al.*, 1987). This publication is divided into two parts, the first discussing the reliability of the Scandinavian suicide statistics, an epidemiological analysis by Lisbet Kolmos, an examination of registration practice and routines by Rolf Hessø and an examination of sources of error in the registration of suicide by Lisbet Kolmos and Elsa Bach. The next section discusses suicide and social integration, in which a pilot study on the degree of social integration in Norway and Denmark has been carried out by Unni Bille-Brahe.

Are there any factors that can protect Norwegians?

In addition to the factors that have been considered, I wish to add something on my own account. The geography of Norway probably plays a role in protecting it against adverse influences from outside. Norway continues to be more of an outpost of Europe than Sweden, Denmark and to some extent Finland. Norway has preserved a rural character, with a fairly widespread pattern of settlement which there have been some efforts to preserve. Norwegian political authorities have consciously counteracted movement away from sparsely populated regions. The Norwegian way of life has perhaps not changed as much from the way it originally was as in other countries. More than anywhere else in Europe the inhabitants of Norway head out into nature in their leisure time, in both summer and winter. This is true of both the urban and rural population, and not least the population of the capital. The inhabitants of Oslo have probably still retained significant contacts in the rural environment. A very large proportion of the Norwegian population have their own cabins and country cottages in the forests, in the mountains or on the shores of lakes, where they spend a great deal of their time. They have not entirely given up their rural traditions, and the original contact with nature has been partly preserved. Maximum use is made of the short summer. There is still enough space for everyone to enjoy the form of outdoor living they want to, and many people spend their leisure time in surroundings where they have a great deal of unspoilt nature to themselves. It is likely that these traditions spring from a close affinity over a thousand years with a tough and demanding nature and a harsh climate. In modern times, however, these very traditions can be an elixir of life in industrial society. The same tendencies could also be said to apply to the other Nordic countries, particularly Sweden and Finland.

The Norwegians are reckoned to be the strictest of the Nordic countries from the moral point of view and also to be the ones with the strongest religious leanings. It is well known that Norwegian policy on illegal drugs has been the strictest in the Nordic region, and the regulations to deal with adverse trends of the time with regard to videos, pornography and violence have also been among the strictest in the Nordic countries. Religion without doubt has a strong hold on the Norwegian population, particularly in areas where people have to struggle against the harshest natural forces: in the west and north. Norwegian politicians always have to take account of the strong religious and moral currents in the country. It is the 'dark coastal strip' – the most strongly religious parts of the country in the south and west coast areas that have traditionally had the lowest suicide rate. The Norwegians also probably live to a greater extent than the other Scandinavians in sparsely populated districts, and have more opportunity for coming into closer contact with each other in small groups and small communities where people are more dependent on each other and live more closely together. The tendency towards moving away has probably been less strong in Norway than in Sweden, and in particular less strong than in Finland.

I believe the best medicine to prevent an increase in the incidence of suicide in Norway will be to succeed in maintaining the whole and unseparated nuclear family as the central basic structure in society, and the decentralised parish and village community. The relatively strict moral attitudes and traditions should not be abandoned. Norms and attitudes which counteract trends towards the break-up of families and communities probably also prevent phenomena such as suicide, drug abuse and criminality. However, there should be compromise on the further development of the welfare society, and large concentrations of population should be discouraged and decentralisation encouraged. Although unemployment has not yet been high in Norway (despite the fact that it has risen significantly whilst this book was being produced), it must be assumed that measures to control unemployment in the long-term will also prevent suicide. Attention should be focused not least on the situation faced by young people and in particular young men. An increasing suicide rate precisely in this group suggests that problems have to be faced here which have not yet been identified.

However, the findings which have been referred to, particularly with regard to suicides in young people, are unfavourable for Norway. They suggest that the trends towards the break-up of Norwegian society are taking place more rapidly than in the other Nordic countries – in other words that the same development that reached the other countries earlier is now occurring in Norway. The situation in which the increase in the suicide rate among the young is now in fact higher than in Denmark and Finland suggests that Norway will reach the traditionally high Scandinavian incidence of suicide within a relatively short time, perhaps before the turn of the century. There is little hope of the national suicide prevention programme in Norway having more of an effect than its equivalents in Finland and Sweden, both of which have made greater progress with their national suicide prevention programmes.

7

Sex, age, marital status and social factors

Sex

It was stated earlier that more men than women commit suicide. In Norway a hundred years ago the ratio was 4:1, as mentioned, whilst today it is 2.8:1, in Sweden 2.4:1 and in Denmark 1.7:1. The ratio continues to be 4:1 in Finland. The change which has taken place is believed to have something to do with developments in the pattern of roles for the sexes. The closer the roles of the sexes come together, the smaller the differences are likely to be in phenomena that are sex-related, such as the incidence of suicide.

Attempted suicide, on the other hand, is most common in women. Overall, women make more attempts at suicide than men. There has been a great deal of speculation about the reasons for this. Considering that men more commonly die when they attempt suicide, it might be imagined that this is related to the fact that men adopt more dangerous and more violent means for committing suicide than women. Firearms are often used by men, for example, but rarely by women. The usual female method of committing suicide is poisoning, using medicines which are most readily available in the home medicine cabinet. These days the drugs in question are antidepressants and sedatives.

The fact that attempted suicides in women are more innocuous is nonetheless unlikely to be due to the lower muscular strength of women or their lack of technical knowledge and skills. To a clinician it appears that women, more than men, use the act of suicide as an aggressive weapon, as a defensive weapon or as a means with which to manipulate their environment. This may be related to the fact that women, more than men, are expected to be careful, restrained and less violent, and perhaps also refrain more from aggressive means of expression in general. They fulfil these social expectations when they are in a desperate situation and consider taking their own lives. They will be more likely to take their aggression out on themselves.

As equality has increased the incidence of attempted suicide among men has tended to increase. What happened in Denmark was that an increase in attempted suicide started to occur in the 1970s, and around 1980 men were in fact in the majority for attempted suicide. It appears that this levelling-out between the sexes was manifested first – and most distinctly – in Denmark, but a gradual trend in the same direction is also being witnessed in other countries.

Age

Suicide in childhood

It is rare for children to commit suicide. Suicide in childhood does occur in Norway, but fortunately they are isolated cases. There has not yet been any clear increase in the suicide rate among children under the age of 15 in Norway. However, an increase of this kind has been clearly registered in the USA, where the suicide rate for children between the ages of 10 and 15 is now two per 100,000 per year. The increase has been so significant in the USA that it has aroused concern, and has led to suicidology having been included in school curricula. Case material from the USA suggests that children who commit suicide are very frustrated individuals who have lacked tenderness, love and affection, or who end up in an insecure situation which drives them to despair. Quite commonly it is the often hopeless situation of the child in connection with the splitting-up of its parents. The material shows that half the children who take their own lives or attempt to do so come from broken homes or from homes with single parents, or from children's homes. Growing up without both parents thus appears to be a risk factor in itself. Over 10% of suicidal children live in children's homes or with foster parents. A statistical increase has been registered in suicides among children in England, Germany, and the first signs of the trend have been observed in Denmark and may be expected to reach Norway. This increase presumably relates to the fact that more children are growing up in insecure family situations and without the closeness and security which a nuclear family, in spite of everything, can provide.

There are other European studies which suggest that perhaps the statistics relating to suicide in children should be viewed with some caution. To most adults, suicide in children is almost unthinkable, and the possibility of a child taking its own life is discounted. It is therefore possible that childhood deaths which really are suicide are registered as accidental deaths. This need not be related to any wish to conceal the suicide, but may be due to no thought being given to the possibility that the accident was intended. No studies have been conducted in Norway which can shed light on this problem.

Suicide in youth

The incidence of suicide has traditionally been low in the younger age group (15–29 years of age), but a sharp rise has been registered in the Nordic region, in the world in general and unfortunately quite specifically in Norway, as already discussed. Attempted suicide has traditionally been very common in this group, particularly among girls, and has usually been connected with the loss or threatened loss of steady relationships as a result of engagement or marriage. The incidence of attempted suicide is also particularly high in this age group today, particularly among women.

Suicide in the elderly

In Norway it is now the over-80 age group which has the highest suicide rate as far as men are concerned, and there is a very distinct predominance of men who commit suicide in the higher age groups (ratio 6:1 of men to women, compared with a ratio of 2.8:1 in the other age groups).

The suicide rates are high for the very old in most western countries. For men in the 75–79 age group, the suicide rate in all European countries is under 100, except in France where it was 101.9 (WHO data bank), closely followed by Czechoslovakia with 91.1. The figures date from 1985. In the 80–84 age group the rate was over 100 in both these countries (132 and 110.3 respectively), and in the over-85 age group it was 158.9 and 112 respectively. However, there were two other countries in which the rate was over 100 in this high age group: West Germany (103.6) and Japan (102.1). In the USA the rate rose with age, except in the very oldest group. The rate for men was 29 in the 65–69 age group, 38.9 in the 70–74 age group, 58.4 in the 75–79 age group, 61.9 in the 80–84 age group and 55.4 in the over-80 age group. The rates with respect to women are fairly steady in these age groups. There are, therefore, major differences in rate between the sexes in the upper age groups, and the higher the age the greater the differences are. The only exception is Japan, where the suicide rates among women increase in line with those for men in the upper age groups. The suicide rate among the elderly has increased in all countries over a ten-year period.

Suicide among those aged over 60 now accounts for a quarter of all suicides in the USA (Richardson, Lowenstein & Weissberg, 1989), and in the Netherlands a third of all suicides (Kerkhof, Visser & Diekstra, 1990). In Japan suicide among women aged over 60 accounts for 45% of all female suicides (Tatai, 1991). Three-quarters of all suicides in the USA among the elderly are committed by men, the rate increasing progressively with age from 31 per 100,000 in the age range 65–74 years, to 46 in the age range 74–84 years, to 50 in the persons over 85.

Divorced, unmarried and widowed people have a suicide rate which in most countries is around three times higher than among married people. Social isolation plays a particularly great role among the elderly.

More violent methods are used in upper age groups, particularly by men. In most western countries it appears that over 85% of the total suicides among the elderly occur by hanging (especially in men), poisoning (especially in women) and drowning. The elderly frequently die by means of 'slower' methods, for example, neglecting themselves, refusing food or drugs, or not complying with treatments. These methods do not appear in official statistics of suicide and it is believed to be one of the most important causes of the underestimation of suicides among the elderly.

The rate of attempted suicide appears to decrease with age, but the ratio between attempted suicide and suicide, which in younger age groups is around 10:1, is closer to 2:1 in the older age groups, suggesting a far higher degree of serious attempts among the elderly with a fatal outcome.

There are many special triggering factors among the elderly. It was believed that the introduction of the old-age pension with increased financial security would reduce the rate. Sainsbury (1963) was able to show that the introduction of old-age pensions in Great Britain did not lead to any such reduction.

The leading factors among the elderly appear to be the feeling of a lack of purpose, retirement, loss of close friends and relations (particularly husbands and wives), moving (particularly from the home to an institution), lack of a network, a reaction of grief and perhaps most of all chronic, painful or terminal illness. But depressive disorders are greatly underestimated and inadequately recognised and treated in the elderly. The same applies to other psychiatric disorders and not least alcohol problems (De Leo & Ormskerk, 1991).

It is estimated that about 80% of elderly people who commit suicide are suffering from a depression which has for half of them lasted for a year; few have been given adequate treatment. Three-quarters of the elderly patients who commit suicide have consulted a physician during the month and one-third during the week prior to the suicide.

Marital status

Suicide is less common among married people, particularly when they have children, than in those who are single, divorced or widowed. Statistics from the USA show that the suicide rate among single men is twice as high as among married men. Among widowers and divorced men it is three and five times higher, respectively, than among married men. The ratio is similar for women, except for the youngest age group (15–24). In this group married women have just as high a suicide rate as unmarried women. Those without children have a higher suicide rate, this applies particularly to women.

For married boys aged 15–19 the suicide rate is 1.5 times higher than for unmarried boys of the same age, and for girls it is 1.7 times higher. This has been interpreted as being due to the fact that marriage at this age has often not been properly thought through and can often be viewed as an escape from an unsatisfactory home situation (Bjerke, 1990).

An attempt at an explanation

It is logical to imagine the explanation for the low rate among those who are married being that marriage provides protection against suicide. This may possibly be connected with the married person having someone to share and discuss his or her problems with, and with the fact that suicide to a greater extent would affect someone else. They also have responsibility for each other, particularly if they have children. The problem of isolation would not arise to the same degree as for those living alone, although it is well known that there are plenty of people who are isolated within their marriage.

On the other hand, selection must be taken into account. It is possible that the same factors have an influence on whether an individual is to remain unmarried, be married, become divorced or commit suicide.

People with relationship problems, an inclination towards isolation and great insecurity in themselves can easily remain single. It is also likely that among those who become divorced, there will be some predominance of people who are less stable and with a greater tendency to develop conflicts in their inter-human relationships and possibly also to evade problems and choose escape solutions. Added to these factors are marital conflicts and divorce itself, which are always stressful. It is difficult for the selection principle to explain the high incidence among persons of widowed status. Here it is reasonable to cite psychological problems, such as loneliness, isolation and economic problems associated with the widowed status. There will obviously be relatively more people of widowed status in the highest age groups, and as we have seen, the suicide rate is particularly high in the 75–80 age group. Physical disorders obviously also occur in the oldest age groups. The great predominance of men in the highest age groups may suggest that it is more difficult for an old man to cope alone.

Social factors

These appear to be of great significance in triggering suicide. The founder of Norwegian sociology, Eilert Sundt, published his classic treatise on mortality in Norway back in 1855. He would without any doubt have been counted as one of the great pioneers of social science if he had written in a world language. He attributed major importance to social conditions in triggering suicide. He laid great emphasis on the responsibility of the community and on the society of which the person who committed suicide was a member. The first person to try to identify the causal factors behind suicide on a more scientific basis was the French sociologist Emile Durkheim, who in 1897 published his famous monograph *Le Suicide* (see later French edition 1912; English translation 1952). This has since become the most widely quoted book on the problem of suicide. There is still considerable interest in it. Durkheim considered suicide to be understandable only on the basis of the society in which the individual lives. He believed that the better an individual is linked to the society or a smaller social or religious group, the lower the likelihood of suicide will be. The more lonely and isolated the individual is, the greater the likelihood of suicide. Durkheim subdivided suicides into four types: egoistic, altruistic, anomic and fatalistic. We discussed the first three earlier (page 20). In fatalistic suicide there is too much control by society, and the individual who is tormented by strict discipline and terror attempts to escape through suicide.

Today, social integration or lack of social integration is regarded as a key factor in the problem of suicide. The term integration is used to mean the membership of and feeling of belonging to various groups of society, for example family, team at work, religious and political groups. I have previously discussed this relationship in our examination of the Scandinavian suicide problem. I have also considered the problem while speaking about the role of age factors and marital status. It is also a factor which goes some way towards explaining why suicide is more common in urban areas, with a greater likelihood of isolation and loneliness, and is less common in rural communities, where people largely feel a greater sense of belonging.

Suicide occurs most commonly at two extremes of the economic scale – among those at the top and among those at the bottom of the socio-economic ladder. This is particularly noticeable in the USA, where the suicide rate is particularly high in the lowest social group, which is considerably worse off than the lowest social group in Norway in relative terms, and among business managers who lead stressful, taxing lives and have responsibility for many jobs and the success of their firms. In the lowest social group people will be found who are unemployed, live in misery, have severe economic problems, move around a great deal and often have problems with alcohol and drug addiction and physical and mental disorders.

Doctors, dentists and pharmacists

This group are considered to have a high suicide rate, which may be linked to knowledge of and access to the means of committing suicide, but may also be linked to an irregular and stressful occupation. It has been shown that women doctors, in relative terms, have a higher suicide rate than male doctors. The reason for this is probably that although female doctors, like other doctors, have a very stressful job and also have to deal with the problems of many other people, unlike male doctors, however, the tasks and responsibilities of the home also await her, with greater responsibility for children and the home and household chores. She thus has more responsibility and work thrust upon her than her male counterparts. In Denmark 50% more suicides have been found among doctors than in the population at large, and the figures are even higher in the

USA. Recent studies from Bavaria (Bämayr, 1983) and Sweden suggest, however, that male doctors do not have a higher suicide rate than equivalent academically trained persons, but that the increased mortality is clear with regard to female doctors. One of the reasons why doctors and other health-care personnel probably have a high suicide rate is that it is a group which is more difficult to treat. Doctors in particular find it more difficult to identify themselves with the role of patient and will tend to reject treatment or discontinue it.

Students

These are another group with a high suicide rate. Suicide is the third most common cause of death among college students in the USA. In Britain it has been shown that the suicide rate varies widely from one university to another. It is particularly high in the old, renowned universities of Oxford and Cambridge but is particularly low in the provincial universities. It is thought that this may be due to the students at the latter having more contact with their families and with society in general, and to the fact that they do not live in such isolation. The level of ambition is higher at Oxford and Cambridge. The families have often also placed particular expectations on these students, who did not have a close relationship within their home environment either. Loneliness, isolation, living in bedsits and a strange environment far from home may have a part to play in the high suicide rate, but there are certainly also economic concerns, concerns about examinations, failing and a fear of not living up to expectations.

Attempted suicide is also more common among students than in a corresponding population of the same age, a finding which also emerges from Nordic studies. There is also an impression in Norway that the suicide rate among students is relatively high. However, no research has been carried out in this area. It is well known in medical circles that medical students working as house doctors are at risk of suicide. This is considered to be linked to the fact that they have led a relatively protected existence as students, without the burden of responsibility which is placed on them when they are on duty and having to hard work as house officers in hospitals or in practice. They have little training in taking quick decisions, which may often have life and death consequences for their fellow humans. Although they have an experienced doctor to back them up, house doctors will be the first to arrive and their decisions may be decisive. This is a tough task for a young and relatively inexperienced person who is also at the stage of establishing himself in terms of family, specialisation and economics.

However, there are studies which indicate that the suicide rate is not higher for students. A survey by the American College Health Association (1980) found a lower suicide rate among students than among non-students (Schwartz & Reifler, 1980). The same finding was made at Alberta University in Canada and in Edinburgh (Platt, 1986). Bjerke (1991) found the same in Norway.

Sailors

A high suicide rate has been observed among sailors. It has been shown in Norwegian surveys that the suicide rate among sailors is three times higher than in a corresponding land-based population (Arner, 1970). Suicide is the second most common cause of death at sea in the Norwegian merchant fleet, and accounts for 15% of fatal accidents. Only death from drowning ranks higher. Most suicides take place at sea, not while the ship is in port. Suicide mortality among sailors is particularly high in the youngest age groups, 15 to 29-year-olds. The first period at sea appears to be particularly high-risk (first-trip boys). Some sailors have traditionally been recruited from among young people who find it difficult to adapt at home and in school, a tradition which has now ceased. The life of a sailor continues to be tough, however, with considerable isolation, little and irregular contact with family, irregular hours of work and not least with ready access to alcohol. In Norway there are fewer and fewer sailors, however, since large parts of the Norwegian merchant fleet have been registered abroad, and lowly paid foreign sailors such as Filipinos have taken over the crewing of Norwegian ships, on which soon only the captains and first mates will be Norwegian.

The unemployed

Many studies, both in Norway and in other countries, have demonstrated a statistical link between unemployment and the occurrence of suicidal behaviour. There are certainly many interrelated factors in the increased incidence of suicide among the unemployed. British studies in particular have shown this. It is the social and psychological consequences of unemployment that appear to be central, and long-term unemployment in particular is a stressful factor. It is important to us humans to be in work, both so that we can feel meaningful and so that we can have our economic needs fulfilled, and not least also to acquire social contacts. Those who become unemployed are often people who had previously found it difficult to assert themselves, who have a low level of education, who perhaps have previously acted on the margins, and who in some cases have also suffered mental problems. Some of the characteristics which predispose people to unemployment also predispose them to suicide: coming from broken homes, leaving home early, having personality disorders, and not least abusing alcohol and drugs.

A Danish study from the 1980s showed that among a group of people who attempted suicide only half as many were in employment as in the general public, and that those who were in work were poorly integrated. Integration in working life was particularly poor among men in the 40–49 age group who attempted to commit suicide. This in turn was in sharp contrast to the high level of integration in this age group generally. There are also studies from Norway which indicate that suicide and attempted suicide occur more commonly among the unemployed. It must be borne in mind, however, that up to the end of the 1980s, Norway was largely spared unemployment. A striking development has been the sharp rise in suicide among the young, which was mentioned earlier. This increase has been sharpest in Norway, and far greater in Norway than in Denmark, in a period when there was no unemployment in Norway, whilst the unemployment rate was relatively high in Denmark. Retterstøl, Hessø & Ekeland (1985) found that of the suicides registered among the younger population in Oslo, none was unemployed. Unemployment is therefore scarcely the sole predisposing factor in itself.

Immigrants, refugees and emigrants

These are groups who are at risk of mental illness in general. Emigrants have a higher suicide rate, both compared with their compatriots back in the old country and natives of the new homeland. In the USA it has been shown, for example, that Swedish immigrants had twice as high a suicide rate as in their homeland, and that Norwegians had three times the rate. The suicide rate among Scandinavian immigrants in the USA shows the same trends as in Scandinavia: a higher suicide rate among Finnish, Danish and Swedish immigrants than among Norwegians. Many factors contribute to the increased incidence of suicide among immigrants and refugees. They have broken out of the group to which they naturally belong, often under difficult circumstances, and they have to cope in new and unfamiliar surroundings, often with a new language and unfamiliar customs, to which it can take a long time for them to adapt. In the long run, constantly having to be newly introduced to people gets them down. The basis for isolation has thus been laid.

Political refugees are a particularly vulnerable group. They have often been through a long process, perhaps involving bugging, imprisonment and torture, and have lived for a long time in a situation in which they have had to be on their guard. In addition, they have had the burden of having to get out of their own country, have perhaps been interned in refugee camps and have faced problems in seeking asylum and applying for residence permits in the new country.

It is particularly during the initial period following the move that there is a high suicide rate among immigrants, refugees and emigrants. However, there are also problems in the second generation, particularly when they come from strange cultures, perhaps with a different ethnic and religious background than the population of the country they have come to. The traditional role which they are expected to fulfil in their old culture may be in sharp contrast to the role they are expected to play in an industrialised society with freer conventions and different norms. Children of immigrants may therefore find it difficult to discover their identity and where they belong, and may encounter conflict situations which can lead to self-destructive acts. The inclination towards suicide among immigrants follows the pattern of the country they come from. In Moslem countries, the inclination towards suicide is low, probably due to religious factors. The suicide rate among the many Turkish immigrants in West Berlin, for example, is lower than in the rest of the population of West Berlin, but appreciably higher than in Turkey.

Military service

This can also cause particular social isolation which is accompanied by a high suicide rate. According to statistics from the USA, the incidence of suicide in the military in peacetime, when the figures are corrected for age and sex, is almost twice that in the general population. It has been assumed that this is linked to the soldiers readily becoming indifferent, not having sufficient challenges to face and viewing their existence as stultifying and of little use. There is little scope for personal initiative and satisfying one's own needs. The incidence of suicide among servicemen falls in wartime, as it also does in the population at large – the suicide rate in the US forces fell to a fifth during the Second World War compared with the period before. This figure has been linked to the aggressive tendencies that suicide often expresses being more easily directed in wartime into directly aggressive outward acts, either into acts of war or into aggressive feelings against the enemy. It can also be imagined that self-destructive tendencies would be channelled into daring operations against the enemy, where death is not recorded as a consequence of suicide but as a consequence of acts of war. It may also be assumed that cohesion in the population in the fight against a common enemy detracts attention from personal problems and conflicts. However, it can also be quite generally expected that the recording of suicide will become less reliable in wartime. The suicide rate among servicemen in Norway in peacetime has been found to be like that in a corresponding non-military population (Hytten & Weisæth, 1989). Bearing in mind that those who enter military service are a positive selection of the population, in that drug abusers, people with personality disorders, etc., are excluded in advance, these are nevertheless findings which suggest that the problems of military service may well be a source of considerable stress. Mehlum (1991) studied attempted suicides among conscripts in the Norwegian armed forces, and did not find any particular increase in the rate from 1968 to 1989. Most of those who attempted suicide had had a difficult childhood, had personality disorders, problems of adjustment or were depressed. Less dangerous methods were used. They were generally dismissed.

Criminals

Criminals have a high rate of both suicide and attempted suicide. Both are probably due to predisposing features in the criminals and the distinctive situation they often end up in. People who become criminals are often people who are emotionally immature, have little control over their urges and have a tendency to give in to momentary impulses without the usual regulatory mechanisms which most people have built into them. They often have little persistence and little ability to work towards longer-term objectives. They often also harbour powerful aggressive feelings, partly against those close to them but not least against society. If they are frustrated, the aggression may in some cases be channelled into acts of violence and in some cases be directed inwards, resulting in attempted suicide and suicide. Both sets of acts exist at the same time. It is quite common for a person confronted with the results of the external aggression, as in murder and acts of violence, to be seized by aggression directed inwards and afterwards commit suicide or attempt suicide. The incidence of attempted suicide in custody cells and prisons is very high. The period spent in custody is the time of greatest risk.

Alongside the factors already mentioned, the high incidence of suicide is certainly also linked to degradation, humiliation and not least the isolation that is experienced in prison and in the cell. It is also linked to the prosecution situation, uncertainty about the future and the prospect of long-term isolation in prison. There may also be some connection with the attempt at suicide serving the purpose of making an appeal, in the hope that the result will be a pardon, being declared unfit to serve a sentence, or a spell in hospital. It is well known that prisoners are capable of undertaking the most grotesque attempts at suicide, for example by swallowing razor-blades, knives or scissors. This often leads to surgery with prolonged spells in hospital.

Here, as elsewhere, it is always difficult to assess how 'seriously' the attempted suicide was meant. The ratio between suicide and attempted suicide in prisons is roughly the same as in the rest of the population. It is during the period spent in custody and during the first phase of imprisonment, after sentence has been passed, that the danger of suicide is greatest. The better and more humane our treatment of criminals can become, the more likely it is that we will be able to reduce the incidence of suicide among inmates.

Suicide in Norwegian prisons over a 35-year period has been analysed by Hammerlin (1992). Over this period, 60 suicides were registered of which 49 (82%) have been committed since 1970 (43 between 1970 and 1989 – see Figure 7.1 – none in 1990, four in 1991 and two in 1992 at the time of writing), which clearly suggests that the extent of the problem is increasing.

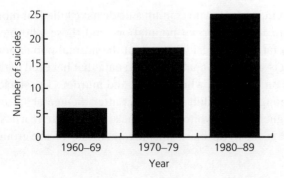

Figure 7.1. Suicide in Norwegian prisons in the three last ten-year periods (from Hammerlin, 1992).

Calculated according to various statistical methods, the rate is in any case around ten times higher than among the population at large. Half of those who committed suicide were 25 years of age or younger and 72% were under the age of 30. All committed suicide in closed institutions – 93% in ordinary cells or in high-security cells. A third committed suicide during the first week, 48% during the first three weeks and 77% during the first three months of imprisonment. This shows clearly that the risk is greatest during the initial period of the time spent in prison. This is in good agreement with international studies. In 75% of cases the method used was by hanging. Those suspected of homicide or attempted homicide were a particularly high-risk group, as were drug abusers and young people sentenced for violent crime. Many were socially marginalised and belonged to multi-problem groups. Hammerlin states that a great deal can be done in prison care to prevent suicide.

Suicide and violence

It is common to find an inverse ratio between suicide and violence – in societies with a high suicide rate, the homicide rate is low. Denmark and Sweden are examples of this. However, in Norway both rates are lower, and in Finland both rates are higher. In the USA, the suicide rate among whites has been high and the murder rate low, whilst among blacks the murder rate has been high but the suicide rate has been low. The situation in the USA is changing. Hendin (1982) states that over the last 20 years prior to the publication of his study, both the suicide rate and the murder rate increased by 300% among white men aged 15–19. For young men, both the suicide rate and murder rate in this group are among the highest in the world.

Hendin states that individuals who commit suicide have killed far more often than the figure for the normal population, and those who have killed others have a far higher suicide rate than the normal population. Hendin states that it is superficial analyses of the data that have led to the views which prevail on black and white suicide and murder. The suicide rate is very high among young adult blacks, but after the age of 45, the suicide rate is far higher among whites. The black murder rate reaches a peak in the same age group as the black suicide rate: the 20–35 age group.

Homosexuals

Homosexuals have a high suicide rate. Isolation, loneliness and difficulty in adjusting are key problems. Selection plays a major role for some groups – personality features have predisposed them to enter these groups. There may be underlying distorted personality developments from childhood, but the psychological situation is also particularly difficult, since the majority in society continue to look down on, reject and despise those who are 'different'. Male homosexuals in particular often have short-term relationships with frequent break-ups and an existence which can easily become rootless. Problems with HIV infection and AIDS affect homosexuals to a far greater extent than other population groups, which is obviously another source of severe stress. Female homosexuals appear to be more readily accepted. For those who are bisexual, special problems can obviously arise if, for example, they are married.

Hendin (1982) refers to his own study of suicide among blacks (1971), in which he found that four out of 12 seriously suicidal black men were homosexual, whilst the percentage of homosexual men in a normal population, both for blacks and whites, is quoted as being 5–10%. He did not obtain equivalent findings for women.

Status integration

The results which have been referred to strongly support Durkheim's hypotheses, which we have also considered during the discussion of the Scandinavian suicide problem. The expression *status integration* is central to suicidology. Durkheim formulated the following postulation: 'Suicide varies in inverse proportion to the integration of social groups.' Following the same line, Gibbs & Martin (1964) examined the statistical link between status integration and suicide in various countries and social groups. They came to the following conclusion: 'The incidence of suicide in a population varies with the degree of status integration in the same population.' The less status integration, the more suicides. This theory is confirmed by the higher suicide rate not only among refugees, emigrants and those without roots, but also among the divorced and separated. To some extent the argument can be used to explain differences in suicide rate between occupational groups and religious groups, between town and country, or parts of a country compared with other parts, and countries in comparison with others. These theories have formed the basis for our analysis of the Nordic differences in suicide rate.

Geographical distribution

The incidence of suicide not only varies between countries but also within the individual country. The situation everywhere is that the suicide rate is higher in urban areas, and the larger the population of the towns and cities is, the higher the rate. The suicide rate is lower in small towns but in turn is higher than in sparsely populated areas. The suicide rate tends to be proportional to the size of the town or city. Within cities a higher suicide rate is usually found in areas with a changing population and in areas with many people in bedsits, people living in boarding-houses and the elderly. The suicide rate tends to be lowest in the more wealthy suburbs with detached houses and economically and socially privileged people who have been able to afford to and have had the opportunity to settle there. Over-representation of suicide in large cities is also assumed to be linked to the likelihood of social isolation and anonymity being greatest there. The suicide rate is high in slum districts in large cities in the West. This is probably due firstly to the miserable conditions the population live under, but also to the fact that these districts attract mentally unstable people who have problems in adjusting, alcohol and drug-related problems and criminal tendencies.

Time of year, day of the week, time of day

Most statistics show that the rate of suicide is lowest in the darkest winter months, increasing gradually towards the spring and usually peaking in May and June. The rate usually drops again from August and September. Figures from Australia suggest that the suicide rate is highest in the last few months of the year, i.e. the time corresponding to spring in the northern hemisphere. No satisfactory explanations for this have been given. However, it has been suggested that people generally live a more isolated life in the winter, and that the isolated person is not confronted with his isolation so much at that time. When the forces of life awaken and people go out again in the spring and summer, the lonely and isolated person will be more likely to be confronted with his isolation. The forces of life then have an almost provocative effect. Hjortsjø (1983) has found with regard to the Scandinavian countries that the months of November, December and February have a significantly lower rate of suicide, whilst

May and August show a significantly higher rate. With regard to days of the week, Hjortsjø showed in the Stockholm study that the number of suicides was considerably lower on Tuesdays than on the other days of the week. There is a close correlation between suicide and the influence of alcohol. Variations in the incidence of suicide according to months and days may relate to the pattern of drinking. It is usually difficult to give precise figures for the time of day when suicide is committed. Most believe that it is the afternoon, evening and night that are the highest-risk times of day.

8

Methods used in suicide and attempted suicide, and warnings

The methods most commonly used in suicide are poisoning, hanging, shooting, drowning and falling from great heights, in the order in which the methods are used at present in Norway. Cutting instruments are also involved in attempted suicide, usually for slashing.

There are clear differences between the sexes. A far higher percentage of women commit suicide by poisoning. Hanging is used to a greater extent by men and shooting almost exclusively by men. Drowning is more evenly distributed. It appears that women have a greater tendency to choose methods in which appearance is preserved better, that is more 'acceptable' methods. In countries where hanging is used as a death penalty for murderers, suicide by hanging has been proportionally rare. This may be due to the method having been connected with a gruesome crime in people's consciences.

The choice of method depends to some extent on opportunities and cultural circumstances. In the USA around half of suicides are carried out by shooting, which may be linked to the fact that firearms are more readily available there. Suicide by gassing oneself is becoming increasingly rare, as fewer and fewer people use gas in the home. The various methods of committing suicide appear to have a fairly equal percentage distribution from one year to another within the individual country.

A combination of more than one method is quite commonly used, for example taking tablets and falling from great heights or drowning. This is a form of double guarantee that the attempt will succeed. The person in question has often drunk a large amount of alcohol beforehand, partly so that the braking mechanisms are kept in check. It is found that alcohol can be detected in the blood of around half those who die by suicide.

In a few cases the person committing suicide takes special precautions to prevent help, for example locking the door or going to a place where the likelihood of being discovered is low. The rule, however, is that there is generally a possibility of help and that not all the options are closed. In around 80% of suicides it is found that other people have been directly or indirectly warned about what is going to happen, and sometimes they are even told the time and place.

A distinction is often made between what are referred to as *determinant* and *indeterminant* methods. Violent methods such as shooting, hanging and falling from great heights are described as determinant methods, because they provide little opportunity for rescue, and also for changing one's mind. People who are mentally ill, particularly the insane, will often choose violent determinant methods. Most attempted suicides are carried out by indeterminant methods, methods which provide some opportunity for rescue. Many suicidal acts are half-hearted acts, with many opportunities for rescue. Often people are expected, a dose is taken which is at the limit or cuts are inflicted which are not particularly deep.

Poisoning is clearly the dominant method of committing suicide among women. Poisoning generally accounts for around a third of suicides. We shall look at the situation in Norway more closely.

Table 8.1 classifies suicides by cause of death as a yearly average for five-year periods up to 1985. Shooting is almost as common a method of suicide in men as poisoning. On the other hand, shooting is very rare among women. The next most common method of suicide used is hanging, which is frequently used by men, but is also used to a considerable extent by women. These methods are followed by drowning. It can be seen from Table 8.1 that drowning is relatively more common among women than among men. Suicide using cutting or stabbing implements is rare, whilst jumping from great heights is slightly more common. Only in around 2% of suicides is the method employed not known.

Figure 8.1 shows how suicide from poisoning has developed in Norway.

As we can see from this graph, the number of suicides from poisoning almost doubled over the period 1970–87. It should be remembered that the suicide rate in Norway also doubled over the same period. Suicide from poisoning has thus maintained its share of suicides. On the other hand, a significant change has occurred with regard to the substances used for committing suicide.

Table 8.1. *Suicide classified by method*

Cause of death	Men[a]							Women[a]				
	Number	%	1966–70	1971–75	1976–80	1981–85	1987	1966–70	1971–75	1976–80	1981–85	1987
Total	649	100	222	272	345	424	486	74	95	128	153	163
Poisoning	183	28	39	62	81	90	113	30	41	56	64	71
Hanging/suffocation	182	28	75	85	98	123	139	16	18	28	36	43
Drowning	49	8	17	23	21	28	24	19	23	22	32	25
Cutting/stabbing implements	21	3	10	9	9	11	14	2	3	3	3	7
Jumping from a great height	20	3	7	11	11	17	12	5	6	9	9	8
Other or no information	11	2	5	5	9	8	6	1	2	6	4	5

Note: [a] Yearly average for each five-year period
(*Source:* Central Bureau of Statistics of Norway, 1987.)

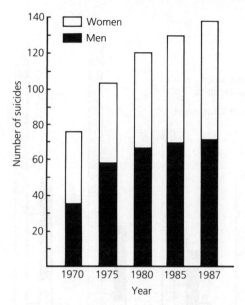

Figure 8.1. Suicide in Norway from poisoning.

Poisoning

Which substances are used for committing suicide? Figure 8.2 shows which groups of drugs were responsible for suicidal deaths from poisoning between 1970 and 1987. This graph shows clearly that barbiturates, which were in general use in 1970, have now almost disappeared from the picture. This is due to the stricter rules which have been introduced on the prescribing of barbiturates and the fact that most barbiturates were taken off the market in 1980. Very few barbiturates are therefore on sale, and there are few barbiturates lying around in medicine cabinets.

There is no detailed recording by the Norwegian Central Bureau of Statistics of the various types of antidepressants used. An analysis was made in conjunction with Finn Gjertsen (1987) against the background of the deaths reported in 1987. This analysis shows the results presented in Table 8.2. Table 8.2 includes 16 cases in which it was not possible to discover which antidepressant had been used. It can be clearly seen from the Table that amitriptyline is the antidepressant most commonly used in suicide, followed by doxepin. Figure 8.3 shows which antidepressants were the most commonly prescribed on the Norwegian market. It can be seen from this chart that one of the antidepressants, mianserin, held a

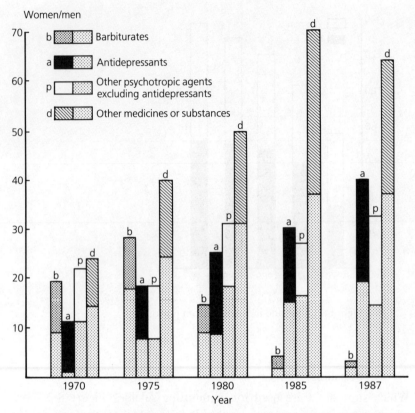

Figure 8.2. Number of deaths in Norway from suicide by solid or liquid narcotic substances (E 950).

Table 8.2. *Antidepressants, main drug used for suicide in 1987*

	Men	Women	Both sexes
Amitriptyline	6	7	13
Doxepin	4	3	7
Imipramine	0	1	1
Trimipramine	1	1	2
Not specified	8	8	16
Total	19	20	39

(*Source:* Central Bureau of Statistics of Norway.)

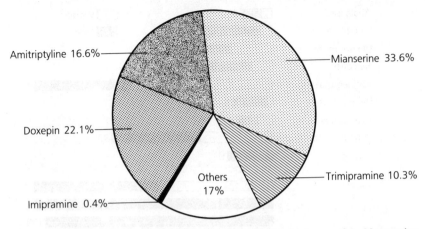

Figure 8.3. Antidepressants, sales in percent on the Norwegian market. (From overall statistics for 1987 of the Norwegian Medicinal depot (Norsk Medisinaldepot))

market share of 33.6% in 1987 but is not mentioned in connection with any deaths.

Morild (1988) has shown the total number of cases of poisoning during the period 1978–87 in Western Norway in a paper from the Norwegian Institute of Forensic Medicine (Rettsmedisinsk institutt) in Bergen (Figure 8.4).

Altogether there were 159 deaths from poisoning, of which 150 were due to medicines. As can be seen from Figure 8.4, antidepressants were the leading drugs used for committing suicide. However, it should be noted that alcohol is the cause of as many deaths from poisoning as all medicines put together.

Antidepressants are found in many homes today. They are also used against deeper depressions, and they are relatively toxic. Fortunately development is now taking place in the field of antidepressants towards drugs which are less toxic, these are referred to as the new generation of drugs, and therefore less dangerous as a means of committing suicide. Antidepressants are taken by patients who are depressed and who therefore pose a greater threat of suicide than others. It is to be hoped that the antidepressants will gradually become less toxic, which will without doubt have a suicide-preventing effect. The substances used to treat mental illness – neuroleptics – are fortunately less effective as a means of committing suicide. They can be used for this purpose, however, particularly in conjunction with other substances.

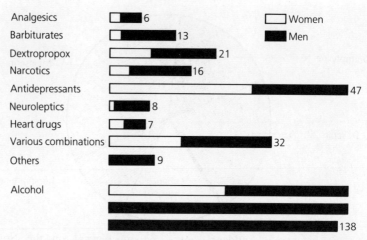

Figure 8.4. The total number of cases of poisoning over the period 1978–87 in Western Norway. Total 159 deaths from poisoning, of which 150 were due to medicines. Over the same period, 138 deaths were caused by alcohol. (From Institute of Forensic Medicine, Bergen (Morild 1988))

Different methods are used in attempted suicide than in suicide. The distribution of methods is also different. In attempted suicide it is chiefly medicines that are used, mostly in the form of tablets. The agents most commonly used are substances which are in fashion at any one time, such as sedatives or hypnotics. These days they are the benzodiazepines, substances such as Librium, Valium, Halcion, etc. Fortunately they are relatively non-toxic. Suicidal attempts with these substances rarely prove fatal if they are taken alone. The barbiturates – the hypnotics – were previously the substances which were most commonly found in medicine cabinets around the home. These were relatively toxic substances which could prove fatal at a dose of 15 to 20 tablets. As we have just seen, these substances have gradually gone out of fashion, and this obviously reduces the danger of this type of medicine proving fatal. On the other hand, antidepressants have become widespread and are thus commonly used in attempted suicide. In the medical department of Ullevål Hospital, in Oslo, Ekeberg *et al.* (1988) shows that antidepressants were the principal means used in attempted suicide. Over the period 1981–83, antidepressants were the principal agent used in 12% of all cases of poisoning admitted to Ullevål Hospital. In 1988 the percentage was the same – 12%. It thus appears that the use of antidepressants as the means of poisoning remained at a relatively stable level in the 1980s, after displacing the barbiturates in the 1970s.

Suicidal attempts are often acts of impulse. This is true not least in the case of poisoning. Studies of people who have attempted suicide show that the act is impulsive in more than two-thirds. The idea of suicide often emerges in the last few minutes before the poisoning takes place. The thought often emerges in connection with a quarrel or a clash with someone the person is close to. The medicine cabinet is there, and for want of anything better, the tablets that happen to be there are swallowed. It has been said that whilst marital conflicts used to be solved by smashing the china, today they are solved via the medicine cabinet.

Other methods

Slashing and cutting the arm, generally the left arm in right-handed people, is a commonly used method. This method rarely constitutes a danger, but often alerts those around the person concerned.

Accidents are without doubt from time to time camouflaged suicide or attempted suicide. There is no doubt that suicidal tendencies are concealed behind some and possibly many road accidents. It is relatively 'acceptable' to end one's life by driving off the road or in a collision, which is registered as an accident and not as suicide. It is 'easier' both on the family and on oneself. It is particularly in cases of driving off the road where the driver has been alone that such thoughts have entered his head. People will generally be careful about involving others in the accident with them, and will thus not undertake the act whilst there are passengers in the car, or in collision with other cars when the lives of strangers may be jeopardised.

More or less unconscious suicidal tendencies are also concealed behind a number of cases of wild driving which result in accidents, not least in the group of people who are described as 'accident-prone' or being 'jinxed'. This type of person is usually characterised by a childish, immature personality structure, with a great deal of 'showing-off' mixed in. Instead of the medicine cabinet, they turn to the car or motorcycle, through which they can express their aggressive feelings and also punish their nearest and dearest. Examples of this are the worker who is criticised by his foreman for not taking care in his work, throws down his tool and leaves the workshop in protest, jumps into his car and drives off at high speed. It is a matter of chance whether an accident will happen or not. Another example is the husband who, after having a row with his wife, gets into the car and drives off at high speed in a reckless manner. There are certainly many causes behind the act: discharge of aggression through the accelerator, suicidal tendency, a belief that 'if anything goes wrong, it'll serve her right', and certainly also a certain satisfaction in performance. The person in question is satisfied if he copes with the potentially lethal situations he puts himself in, and accepts the right solution if it comes. It creates a discharge which other forms of attempted suicide also produce. Fate has to decide. A car accident is often preceded by a crisis situation at work or in marriage. However, studies in the USA (Tabachnick, 1967) suggest that no more than 5% of car accidents have anything to do with the problem of suicide.

Warnings

Suicide generally comes as a shock to relations, friends and acquaintances. However, most have given a hint or a warning of what is going to happen – three out of four doing so. Most people who attempt suicide and do not succeed have also indicated their intentions to others. It is found, however, that around the same percentage of ordinary psychiatric patients who do not attempt suicide have also expressed suicidal thoughts to those around them. On the other hand, it appears that suicidal threats communicated to others are relatively uncommon among non-psychiatric patients.

Most people who allude to their suicidal plans do so in several ways. The hints are often indirect. This may be in the form of preparing a will, arranging what is to be done with capital, actions which can provide useful hints. The most common forms of communicating, in order of frequency, are: statements concerning thoughts about taking one's own life, that it would be better if one was gone, that one wishes to die, that life has no purpose. The people to whom these allusions are made are first of all the husband, wife or partner, followed by relations, friends and the doctor. It is noted that the doctor comes a long way down the list of those to whom the suicidal thoughts are intimated. However, the doctor is the one who comes next after those with whom the person is in closest contact. The message is very often given to a person with whom one is in conflict and towards whom one harbours aggressive feelings.

It is important to note that suicidal threats should be taken seriously. Many people who attempt suicide, and particularly people who succeed in their attempts, leave behind letters or messages, usually to close relations. Feelings of aggression or love are usually expressed towards one or more of those close to the person. Thoughts of revenge are often expressed, as are depressive thoughts and thoughts about death. The person committing suicide is surprisingly often obsessed with what will happen after he dies. He draws up plans for his nearest and dearest and issues guidelines. It is as though he wishes to be involved and have a say in what will happen afterwards. It is generally clear that the person committing suicide wishes through the message left behind to induce certain feelings in those who survive him and who are close to him.

As we now know, attempted suicide is a desperate cry for help. The person in question has usually carefully hinted beforehand through intimations and threats. In the attempted suicide he cries louder. If he succeeds in taking his life, something he often does not really want to do, but feels compelled to, he nevertheless does not abandon the wish to communicate further. He therefore directs the letter to the person or persons he wishes had listened to him before.

Suicide notes

In many cases the person who commits suicide leaves behind a note, usually addressed to key people close to him or her, such as the husband or wife, parents, etc., expressing either aggression or consolation. It is striking to what extent people who take their own lives are obsessed by the consequences of doing so, and also wish to have something to say about how things are arranged in the future. A motive of revenge often plays a part. As mentioned in the description of the cultural history of suicide, there was often a revenge motive in suicide in what are referred to as primitive cultures. People took their own lives 'over the head of the enemy' so that difficulties could be put in the path of the enemy later.

The following are some typical examples of suicide letters, and some examples from suicide letters from the Oslo study (Retterstøl *et al.*, 1985) discussed in chapter 5.

> Dear Kari, I'm sure you know as well as I how fond I am of you. I have always loved you. Everything could have been fine if you had only understood me. What I am now doing is not something that comes easily. You know I made mistakes, which I have regretted and asked your forgiveness for. You know I promised never to do it again, and that I would do everything in my power to make it right again. You know that I wanted to start afresh at home and do everything so much better for you and Ragnhild and John (the children). But you refused to let me come back home again. Time after time I tried, but you were uncompromising. So there is no other way out for me. This is the only one. I

hope you will look after the children well and tell them that Dad was not so bad really. The only annoying thing is that I have just bought that damned expensive car. You can sell it. You are in any case better off now than when you got married seven years ago. Now your worries will be over. I know you have been hoping for this for a long time. I am not mad, I am just fond of you.

Farewell for ever.   Yours, Petter.

Another letter:

My dear wife. I have always been a mistake. I can see that I do not fulfil my obligations towards my wife and children. I am therefore doing what I have always done, choosing the easiest solution. I am leaving you to cope with everything else. But with the insurance payout you will receive, you will manage well enough. Perhaps we shall meet again in a more peaceful place than here on earth.

In the survey of young suicides conducted in Oslo (Retterstøl *et al.*, 1985; see chapter 5), which covered 148 young people (110 men, 38 women) who committed suicide, 32 (17 men; 15 women) had written suicide notes. Suicide notes were therefore approximately three times as common from women, since the suicide rate was three times greater for men. Most letters were addressed to the father or mother. Contrary to expectations, most suicide notes were friendly in nature and expressed gratitude to the parents for what they had done for them. Many also had a religious content and expressed the hope that God would forgive them, and that they would see their family again in Heaven. All the notes were short. Some examples are reproduced here:

I cannot carry on living, dear Mum and Dad. God forgive me. I am nothing to mourn over.

Mother and father. Thanks for everything. You were very kind. I have had problems with my nerves since my studies. Thanks for everything.

Nobody likes me. I am not insane, but I am miserable. I wish to die. Didn't feel any happiness.

Hello everybody. I cannot take any more pain and illness. I've asked God and received forgiveness.

Now I have to do it. Damn it. It's time to put an end to all this nonsense. I've put if off and put it off, and I now I am going to do it.

9

Suicide in physical illness and in general hospitals

Physical illness is an important predisposing factor for suicide. Percentages of between 20% and 40% of cases in which physical illness has played an important role are usually quoted. In an analysis of suicides in London, for example, it was found that cancer occurred 20 times more commonly in a group of those who had committed suicide than in a corresponding normal population. Physical illness is generally recorded significantly more rarely in cases of attempted suicide than in cases of suicide. Physical illness is recorded more frequently in percentage terms as a cause in men than in women. Olafsen (1983) has shown in an analysis of Norwegian figures that there is some predominance of suicide among cancer patients, relatively more among women than men, whilst elderly men as a group are particularly at risk. The risk is particularly high in the first 12 months after the diagnosis has been made. The degree of malignancy is a significant factor, as is age.

The fact that physical suffering has been so often recorded as a cause of suicide may relate to the age factor. Physical illness, like suicide, occurs more commonly among the elderly. Sainsbury (1955) reported that serious physical diseases were associated with 35% of the cases of deaths by suicide in the elderly above 60 years, 27% in those between 40 and 59 years and 10% in younger people. Dorpat, Anderson & Ripley (1968) found still higher percentages, 70, 50 and 13% respectively. The link between physical illness and suicide also appears logical. In some people it is hopeless and painful physical diseases, such as cancer, where the outcome is already decided and the patient shortens his suffering on his own initiative. Physical illness weakens the individual's general and mental powers of resistance, resulting in a feeling of inadequacy and depression. Suicide follows in the wake of depression. For many people life loses its meaning if they cannot continue working or fulfilling a social function. In severe and protracted physical illness, financial worries, worries over the work situation, the family and the future follow. During a period of convalescence following, for example a physical illness or an operation, strength is often low, as is courage, whilst worries are correspondingly many and great. It is assumed that the reason why physical illness leads to suicide more commonly in men than in women is that helplessness and passiveness in connection with disabling illness in our culture is accepted less well by men. The financial and social consequences can also be greater for them, at any rate in present-day society.

Chronic pain can also be difficult to withstand, and demands a great deal of mental energy and therefore takes away resources. Fatigue after protracted infections, anaemia or poor diet do the same. Limited ability to move can make it impossible for a sick or ageing person both to meet the requirements of daily life and make contact with the world around, and both result in a negative impact on the person's capacity for reasonable mental function. Physical illness can also affect the functions of the brain.

We must be aware that even apparently minor physical illnesses can be the starting-point for problems and worries and thus create gloom in the existence of many people.

It is therefore not just in psychiatric hospitals that the danger of suicide is great. Suicide and attempted suicide are not rare in general somatic hospital wards either. This is assumed to relate partly to the increased suicidal tendency in physical illness. It is also connected with anxiety about unknown phenomena such as examinations, operations, courses of treatment etc. Many people also feel a sense of isolation in a large general hospital with a lot of comings and goings. The individual is dehumanised. The geographical location of the hospital may also be such that daily contact with the family is broken. In addition, many patients whose main illness is in fact a psychiatric disorder are admitted to general hospitals. The psychiatric disorder, for example depression, can easily be overlooked, or the treatment of this disorder may be deferred until a general examination has been completed. In a very busy hospital ward, in which doctors and nurses are fully occupied, a potentially suicidal patient can easily feel overlooked and ignored, consider his situation to be even more hopeless, and feel that he might as well put an end to it all. However, what is needed to prevent suicide in general hospital wards, is the same as we shall see is needed in psychiatric institutions: alert, well-trained and understanding staff who relate well to each other and to the patients.

10

Suicide in psychiatric illness

There is a great predominance of death from suicide among psychiatric patients in comparison with the population at large. There is also a great preponderance of attempted suicides in psychiatric illnesses. This may sound obvious and appear to be a circular argument, since many will regard suicide and attempted suicide as an act which in itself is so abnormal that it is an expression or symptom of a psychiatric illness. It is reckoned in the statistics that around a third of those who commit suicide have had a mental illness or severe personality disorder of such a nature that they have been hospitalised. This was also the case in the group of young people committing suicide who were analysed in Oslo over the seven-year period 1975–81 referred to earlier in this book. However, the two-thirds who were not admitted to psychiatric institutions beforehand were not healthy and harmonious people. Retrospective studies, that is, studies backwards through life, show, on the contrary, that many have encountered difficulties with themselves over a number of years, without having been regarded as psychiatric patients.

Over half of those who commit suicide have not been defined as psychiatric patients. However, it is found that two-thirds of them have consulted a doctor during the last six months prior to the act, usually complaining of physical symptoms. The Danish psychiatrist Grete Pærregaard (1963) studied the life-histories of 1470 people who committed suicide. She found that psychiatric illnesses were consistently characteristic of the cases studied. Only in 124 was the suicide unexpected, without the person's relatives having noticed signs of illness beforehand. However, half of these were alcoholics. She concludes that 'if these are deducted, only 68 cases remain out of the 1470 suicides where there is no information on signs of previous mental illness, possibly due to insufficient information.'

Previous illnesses are also common among those who attempt suicide. The incidence of mental illness in the cases studied varies from 4% to 53%. In a more recent study in Sweden, Beskow (1979) largely confirmed Pærregaard's findings.

Psychiatric illnesses with the greatest danger of suicide

Depression

The psychiatric illnesses which most often lead to suicide and attempted suicide are those which fall under the heading of depression. Depression is a collective term for a number of conditions in which the most important symptom is lowered mood. The danger of suicide is particularly high in *melancholia*-type depression. These patients have low self-esteem and a great feeling of guilt and self-accusation. They usually find it difficult to get things off their chest, are inhibited, may find it difficult to get on with others and also to get themselves moving when they are in a period of deep depression. At the same time, they may be overactive and agitated. The condition is often accompanied by physical symptoms, such as poor appetite, constipation, sleeping difficulties, etc. The depression may be so severe that it completely colours the person's experience of himself and those around him, and the patient may develop delusions about having committed the sins of the whole world and being the cause of all the misery in the world, being even worse than, for example Satan. A condition like this is one of the worst types of torment a person can suffer. Life appears to be a heavy burden, meaningless and directly harmful both to oneself and to others. It is, therefore, not odd for suicide and thoughts about suicide to occur. All clinical experience shows that the danger of suicide is not greatest when the depression is at its deepest. In melancholic depression the individual is often too inhibited to undertake such a positive act as suicide and attempted suicide. The danger of suicide is greatest when the patient is on the way out of the depression, and initiative starts to return. The danger is also great before the bottom of the depression has been reached.

In earlier times depression could last between six months and a couple of years. The depression then generally passed over, if the patient survived. These days patients rarely descend into such deep depressions, since we have effective antidepressants which make the depression phase less deep and in particular considerably shorter. However, the risk of suicide also exists, particularly on the way up after antidepressant medication has been started. Unfortunately, the antidepressants are generally also effective ways of committing suicide. It is therefore usually best to leave it to the family to hand out the medicines to the patient, who himself should not have them in his possession whilst he is in the most depressive phase. Antidepressants have now come onto the market which are significantly less toxic (e.g. the tetracyclic drug mianserin, which is significantly less toxic than the most commonly used antidepressants, which are tricyclic moclobemide and fluvoxamin).

The danger of suicide is also great in other types of depression, such as the mild forms of depression triggered in connection with mental problems, the depressive neuroses or the more severe forms of depression triggered in connection with mental difficulties and crises – *reactive* depression. These conditions have generally arisen following difficulties and disappointments in a situation which the person in question cannot find a viable way out of. Antidepressants are also used in these conditions, although with slightly less effect. Psychotherapy is more important. It is necessary to be aware of the danger of suicide in the treatment of these apparently milder forms of depression.

Schizophrenia

Schizophrenics quite commonly commit suicide. The danger is greatest in the initial phase of the illness, when the feeling of identity is wavering, when the patient feels that threatening forces from outside are overwhelming him and a catastrophe is approaching. Internal commands to commit suicide may also be experienced, and ideas of persecution may occur which cause the patient to take steps to escape the persecutors, e.g. by jumping out of a window or throwing himself in front of a train.

Suicide can be triggered in connection with psychotherapy (conversational therapy) for schizophrenic illnesses, where the initial insight the patient gains overwhelms him to such an extent that he cannot see any solution other than suicide. In recent times the danger of suicide in schizophrenics has increased. There are fewer asylum patients today who live a regressive existence in hospital. Instead we have a number of schizophrenic patients who achieve a more or less successful improvement, being able to function outside of the hospital, but not living up to the expectations they had previously set for themselves in relation to work and education. They often follow a marginal existence, perhaps having to go into hospital from time to time, and living a protected life which may be very frustrating. Suicide in schizophrenics is often carried out by violent means. On rare occasions other people may also be taken into death, usually very close members of the family such as parents, partners or children. However, it is more common for such family suicides to be seen in cases of melancholia, because the patients then wish to protect those dear to them against the accidents that are about to happen and therefore involve them in their suicides.

Case material from Norway has shown that patients with functional psychoses (schizophrenia, affective mental illnesses, reactive psychoses) have a suicide rate which is around 20 times higher than that in the general population (Dalgard, 1966; Noreik, 1966). The same excess mortality rate has been shown for paranoid psychoses (Retterstøl, 1966; Retterstøl & Opjordsmoen, 1990). Retterstøl & Opjordsmoen (1990) monitored a group of patients, admitted initially with paranoid psychoses, for a period of as long as 22–39 years. The suicidal tendency was greatest during the first few years, and then declined slightly with the passage of time. Patients with hypochondriac delusions were particularly at risk.

Personality disorders

The danger of suicide is also great in those with personality disorders, such as abnormal personality, psychopaths or sociopaths. These are people who, often since childhood, have shown deviant behavioural traits and have generally been in opposition to everything and everyone. Their personality structure is usually characterised by immaturity. They find it difficult to work towards long-term aims. They seek more instantaneous satisfaction of their drives and needs. Lack of inhibition and restraint tends to characterise these people. In adversity and situations they cannot find a way out of, particularly if the opportunity for natural aggressive outward reaction does not present itself, the aggressiveness may be turned against themselves. Suicide or attempted suicide may then be the instantaneous reaction. A suicidal act and an aggressive act towards others may occur at the same time. It is known that the suicide rate is high in prisons. This is partly due to the type of personality described often being found among criminals.

People with a 'hysterical' personality structure also commit suicide, but in particular undertake attempted suicide. They are people who have a tendency to make themselves the object of attention, who would like to be at the centre, who are obsessed with themselves. This personality type is often also characterised by immaturity and infantility. The attempted suicide often has a distinctive function of an appeal for this personality type, but the danger of suicide must not be neglected for this reason.

Attempted suicide is also seen in connection with what is known as the *abnormal single reaction*. This refers to a brief mental reaction which, with regard to symptoms, is of such a nature as to qualify for the designation mental illness, but which pass over in the course of one day. In such a condition a feeling of panic can develop, with internal tension built up over a long time, and in this desperate situation suicide is quite possible.

These days we often see what are known as 'borderline conditions' in psychiatry, which are to be regarded as personality disorders with an increased readiness to react psychotically. Borderline conditions are usually seen in younger people who have difficulties with their identity and have what we call a 'weak ego', with a poor ability to integrate with the world around and a poor ability to set limits. They find it difficult to make arrangements for the longer term, often undertake acts of impulse and usually have a chaotic image of themselves. They easily become bored, tire quickly, have changeable moods and are unpredictable. But they are stable in their instability. They find it difficult to establish deep interhuman relationships and are often regarded as superficial. They have usually grown-up in difficult circumstances, with instability, changeable relationships with authority and inadequate setting of limits. This type of person easily develops drug problems. Many young drug abusers belong to this category. The danger of suicide is particularly great in this group of people, who can also easily develop psychotic phenomena, often of a schizophrenia-like nature. The condition can go on to develop into schizophrenia, usually lasting only a brief time, but relapses can occur. The danger of suicide is present both outside of and during the psychotic phases.

Organic and senile brain disorders

These also show an excess mortality rate from suicide. The link here is probably that the person falls short of the mark and suffers frustration in relation to his previous resources and the expectations he had of himself.

Crisis situations

In many people suicidal thoughts may arise in connection with sudden crisis situations. Actual or threatened losses, such as for example, the death of a close relative, bankruptcy, the threat of financial ruin, or confiscation of driving licence, can induce severe states of anxiety or internal unease which make the person concerned lose his overview and control of the situation, and he may then find it difficult to control his impulses.

Panic disorders are states of anxiety marked by panic that often occurs in bouts, and which in more recent diagnostic systems are diagnosed as a separate disorder which occurs in 1–2% of the population. The disorder occurs most commonly in women, and is closely related to depression. Antidepressants usually help. It is also necessary to be attentive to the danger of suicide in these states.

Mental disorder in the elderly

An old person generally has fewer resources and may therefore find it difficult to deal with his problems, both illnesses and problems in his life, and can lose control. There is often at the same time loneliness, difficulty in coping with the demands of everyday life, physical disorders, difficulties with relatives or those living in an old people's home, change of home or being placed in an institution. Great sensitivity must be shown towards the elderly person who sees changes taking place in his life situation. They often say little themselves beforehand. It is therefore important to listen to information from relatives.

Suicidal behaviour is often different among the elderly than among the young. The communication of thoughts is more sparse, suicidal attempts may appear to be poorly planned and not dangerous, but the suicide itself can be quite brutal. Suicide by hanging, shooting or jumping from a great height is not uncommon in the elderly. More elderly people die from their suicidal acts than young people. Suicide and age has been discussed in chapter 4.

In recent years there has been an increase in the suicide rate among the very old in Norway, but the suicide rate among the elderly has increased, in relative terms, less than among the other age groups. In many European countries the suicide rate in the elderly is increasing more than in Norway. Suicide in the elderly was the main topic for discussion at the congress of the International Association for Suicide Prevention in 1991.

Abuse of alcohol and drugs

Both suicide and attempted suicide occur significantly more commonly among abusers of alcohol and drugs than in the corresponding general population. The mortality rate from suicide in this group is between 8 and 80 times higher than might be expected in the general population. The death rate from suicide is very high among young drug abusers. There is scarcely any other group of people who have a higher suicide rate than these. In the study by Retterstøl *et al.* (1985) on suicide among young people in Oslo aged between 15 and 29, it was known that a third of them were suffering from alcohol or drug-related problems. In half the young people examined alcohol or addictive drugs were detected in the blood. It has also been shown in a Norwegian study that 1–2% of young drug abusers who have been treated in hospital die each year from suicide or poisoning.

It is not so remarkable that suicide and attempted suicide are so common among abusers, both of alcohol and drugs. It is probably partly due to these people, through their abuse, getting into many complicated situations out of which they are unable to find a way. It also partly relates to the difficult social situation in which they find themselves. In the long run, many close relationships of the alcoholic fail – marriage, job and family life, future prospects become poor, and suicide appears logical. The young drug abusers have often dropped out of society so early in life that they have never entered working life, and naturally enough they will compare themselves with other young people and find they have failed badly.

The high incidence of suicide in these groups is probably also linked to the personality traits which predispose them both to drug and alcohol abuse and to suicide or attempted suicide. In the same way that drug or alcohol abuse can be an expression of the tendency of the abuser to run away from his problems instead of solving them, the attempted suicide or suicide is often an expression of the same thing. Instead of facing the difficult situation and preparing for a more long-term solution, the short-term solution of running away from the whole thing is chosen. The emotional immaturity which often characterises the alcohol and drug abuser is often also characteristic of the person who attempts suicide. In addition, the control mechanisms are weakened under the effect of alcohol or drugs. The normal objections to the act do not emerge.

Studies have been published in the USA containing convincing evidence of the link between alcoholism and suicide, not least from the St Louis group led by Murphy & Robin (1967), Murphy *et al.* (1969). Murphy & Wetzel (1990) have shown that the life-time risk of suicide is around 2% for untreated and outpatient-treated alcoholics in the USA. For alcoholics who have at some time received hospital treatment, the life-time risk was calculated as 3.4%. Murphy (pers. comm., 1992) has identified eight risk factors which are of particular significance for suicide among alcoholics.

How often does mental illness occur in suicide and attempted suicide?

Most sources suggest that around a third of those who commit suicide have a verified mental illness. Of those who attempt suicide, the percentages range from as low as 4% to 53%. This percentage will obviously depend on which patients are studied and also on the diagnostic guidelines followed.

11

Suicide in psychiatric institutions

Increased incidence

The significantly increased danger of suicide among psychiatric patients also suggests that the risk of suicide must be relatively high in the treating institutions which care for psychiatric patients. It is indeed so, despite active efforts to reduce the danger. Studies from Norway by Hessø & Retterstøl (1985) have shown a clear increase in the mortality rate from suicide in Norwegian psychiatric institutions from 1955 onwards. An analysis of deaths from suicide in psychiatric hospitals in Norway is presented in Table 11.1.

Table 11.2 shows the number of suicides per 100,000 patients per year in psychiatric hospitals in Norway over five-year periods from 1930 to 1984. Here again there is a clear rise. Table 11.3 shows the number of suicides in Norwegian psychiatric hospitals per 100,000 first-time admissions and total admissions over five-year periods from 1930 to 1985. A significant increase in the number of admissions to hospitals and a significant drop in the number of in-patients in hospitals over the same period can be seen. However, if suicides in relation to 100,000 first-time admissions are counted rather than the total number of admissions, the numbers vary.

The increase is particularly great if the absolute figures are considered. Whilst the total number of deaths from suicide over an 18-year period from 1937 to 1954 in Norwegian hospitals was 59, the number over the corresponding period from 1955 to 72 was as high as 219. A corresponding increase occurred for deaths resulting from accidents. The total of suicides and accidents was 149 in the first period and 556 in the last period.

Table 11.1. *Absolute number of registered suicides in Norwegian psychiatric hospitals over five-year periods from 1930 to 1984*

5-year period	Registered suicides in psychiatric hospitals
1930–1934	24
1935–1939	26
1940–1944	19
1945–1949	12
1950–1954	14
1955–1959	35
1960–1964	50
1965–1969	71
1970–1974	108
1975–1979	122
1980–1984	90

Table 11.2. *Suicides per 100,000 patients per year in Norwegian psychiatric hospitals reported over five-year periods from 1930 to 1984*

5-year period	Suicide per 100,000 patients
1930–1934	74
1935–1939	76
1940–1944	53
1945–1949	32
1950–1954	35
1955–1959	84
1960–1964	120
1965–1969	169
1970–1974	277
1975–1979	359
1980–1984	373

The trend is clear and leaves no room for doubt: since 1955 a marked and continuous increase has taken place in the suicide rate in Norwegian psychiatric hospitals. The same development has been seen in Sweden. There too, there has been a clear increase since 1955, as Figure 11.1 shows. Results have also been presented from individual institutions in Norway which show clearly the increasing incidence of suicide in recent years. Alnæs (1989) in an article on suicide under psychiatric treatment gives an account of the distribution of 23 suicides at the Psychiatric Clinic in Vinderen over a 30-year period (1959–88), see Figure 11.2.

Table 11.3. *Suicide in Norwegian psychiatric hospitals per 100,000 first-time admissions and total admissions, over five-year periods from 1930 to 1984*

5-year period	Suicide per 100,000 first-time admissions	Suicides per 100,000 total admissions
1930–1934	399	265
1935–1939	369	228
1940–1944	261	146
1945–1949	149	81
1950–1954	186	96
1955–1959	394	190
1960–1964	389	170
1965–1969	519	205
1970–1974	647	247
1975–1979	653	244
1980–1984	693	205

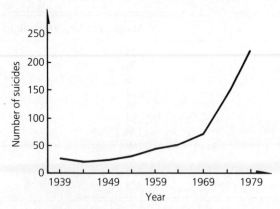

Figure 11.1. Number of suicides at psychiatric institutions in Sweden.

Corresponding findings have been reported from other countries. Hessø (1977) has been able to show the same development in the other Scandinavian countries. Wolfersdorf, Vogel & Hole (1985) showed that there is an increasing tendency towards suicide in psychiatric institutions, not just in Scandinavia but also in Western Europe generally, such as in for example, the former West Germany, Belgium, the Netherlands and Switzerland. In his study he describes a total of 75 scientific studies of this topic in Europe.

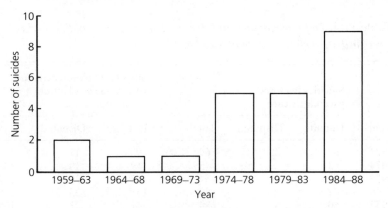

Figure 11.2. Distribution of 23 suicides at the Psychiatric Clinic in Vinderen over a 30-year period (1959–88).

It appears that suicides in psychiatric hospitals are distributed according to age categories fairly similar to the population elsewhere. Half are single. In the West German case material (Wolfersdorf *et al.*, 1985), as many as 68% lived alone, that is were single, divorced, separated or immigrants. Most suicides in institutions take place during the course of the second to fifth stays in the institution. In the study referred to above only 16% of suicides happened during the first admission. They are often long-term patients, the disorder having on average lasted 12 years. Schizophrenia accounted for over half of the cases covered by the study.

There has been much discussion of this increase in suicide in psychiatric institutions in Sweden. Whilst a total of 65 suicides were registered in psychiatric institutions during the period 1930–34, the figure for the period 1975–79 was as high as 335. It is emphasised from Sweden in particular that there is significant under-recording, because suicide which has taken place immediately after a discharge will not be registered as having taken place in hospital. Beskow (1987) has been able to show that the number of suicides committed immediately after discharge is significantly higher than the number of suicides reported in the psychiatric hospitals. Suicide immediately after discharge is therefore a very important and key group. This suggests that patients are discharged too early or that their discharge is not prepared well enough.

Table 11.4 shows clearly how the suicide figures in closed psychiatric wards increase substantially when the registration period is moved by a week and covers the first week after discharge in addition to the active period of admission.

Table 11.4. *Definite suicides and disputed cases among patients who were under psychiatric care in Sweden 1973–79*

Year	Suicides in closed psychiatric care			Suicides in closed care and within one week after discharge		
	Definite	Disputed	Total	Definite	Disputed	Total
1973	67	2	69	90	17	107
1974	43	2	45	119	19	138
1975	50	4	54	117	30	147
1976	72	8	80	153	33	186
1977	80	4	84	141	27	168
1978	61	4	65	125	30	155
1979	72	4	76	182	36	218
Total	445	28	473	927	192	1119

In a study from Denmark (Linder & Wand, 1988) it was shown that there is a clustering of suicides around the time of actual admission and the time of discharge, with a particularly sharp increase during the first week thereafter. These authors also pointed out that suicides occurred particularly in open wards.

Of 522 suicides registered during the period 1979–82, on the island of Funen (population 450,000) in Denmark, 44 admitted psychiatric patients were in institutions, nine were day-patients, 24 were patients treated on an out-patient basis and 40 were in the period immediately following discharge. They show clearly that for those discharged it was the first week which carried the highest risk. As many as 40% of the suicides in the period following discharge from psychiatric hospital occurred during the course of the first week, the remaining 60% during the second to twelfth weeks, and it is noted that the incidence was approximately equal in each of the weeks between the second and twelfth weeks.

Possible explanations for the increased incidence
Changed composition of patients and circulation

We assume that this increase is partly connected with the significantly increased circulation of patients in psychiatric hospitals and partly with a sharp increase in at-risk groups in hospital, such as drug and alcohol abusers. The increase becomes significantly lower if account is taken of the fact that psychiatric hospitals today make the acquaintance of a far larger and more broadly composed set of clients. The number of drug and alcohol abusers for example has increased 20-fold over the same period. This category of patients is the one at most risk of suicide. It appears that the group who take their own lives come from patients for whom the prognosis is relatively gloomy. In the study by Wolfersdorf *et al.* (1985), it was shown that around two-thirds of the patients who took their own lives in psychiatric hospitals in southern Germany were regarded as patients with a poor prognosis and with little likelihood of achieving results from attempts at psychotherapy. Many of these patients had also scored highly in tests with respect to hopelessness and resignation.

Changed methods of treatment and attitudes

The increased incidence of suicide in psychiatric hospitals probably also has some connection with the changed treatment procedures and attitudes which have been adopted in these hospitals during this period. New medicines have come onto the market. They are quite effective both on psychoses and in deeper depressions, but do not effect a radical cure. Active environmental therapy and psychotherapy methods give patients an insight into their illness which they did not previously have, but which can also be hard to take.

Psychotherapy of schizophrenics is a difficult method of treatment, which should be exercised by particularly experienced and capable psychotherapists. These will also know that they need to be relatively less ambitious with the therapy than they are accustomed to being in the treatment of neurosis. It is essential to set to work cautiously and often dampen the expectations the patient, and not least relatives of the patient, have. It is often necessary to make do with a result that is some way away from a cure, but where the clinical – and also social – situation has been significantly improved. Many patients have to be confronted with the fact that an improvement has taken place but that a situation has developed where they cannot be classified as either well or ill. They may be too well to be treated in a psychiatric institution or for continued long-term residence there, but they may also be too ill to cope in a society with the demands that are made today. They often have to make do with marginal work and housing situation, that is with sheltered jobs or homes. It may be quite a terrifying experience for a person who has had great hopes of himself and his future life, and of whom the world around has also had great expectations, to discover that the final result will be an existence with some degree of disability. Accepting this proves to be difficult for the patient and his family, and also for the therapist.

The liberal attitudes in psychiatric hospitals have certainly played a part. It is likely that some increase in suicide is part of the price we have to pay for the open-door policy and for the more humane and democratic methods of treatment we have today. Attention in recent times has shifted away from safety and control measures to human contact, increased activities and more pleasant conditions. In new environmental therapy wards, the situation is often that administrative responsibility for the patients has to some extent been democratised, so that it is not the chief physician but often less experienced physicians who run the ward, who take decisions on patients' home leave and plan of treatment. These are easily affected by the environmental staff, who are often younger and less experienced people and who have a tendency to prefer freedom and liberalism over compulsion and restrictions. Safety measures are probably transferred to a greater extent to groups with less experience and training. Although formal responsibility for the ward and the individual patient remains in the hands of the chief physician, this responsibility in the present situation will be more difficult to tackle for a superior. It necessitates very good and close cooperation with the environmental therapy staff in all cases. This is probably something that can be achieved by introducing what are referred to as contacts for each individual patient, that is people the patient can relate to throughout his stay.

The lower degree of continuity among the attending staff may also play a part. Working hours for employees have been greatly reduced in recent years, and further reduced for those on shift-work. For doctors, the change in working conditions has lead to a great deal of time-off in lieu. This means that the doctors are away from the ward more and are less constantly present than they used to be. The same situation also applies to nurses and other occupational groups. With more changes in both treating and environmental therapy personnel the continuity of treatment is easily disturbed. It is known from the past that holidays and leave for the therapist is always a high-risk time, for which the patient must be prepared. Absences of this kind are now increasing, and it is not always possible to find sufficiently good replacements.

A situation which has arisen in many European countries particularly since the mid-1980s is that of the major administrative shake-ups taking place in the mental health service. Hospitals and wards take over sectorised areas of responsibility, and patients no longer belong to the same wards or treatment institutions as before. In Oslo this has happened to an extreme degree in recent years in connection with sectorisation. The hospitals had been sectorised over a ten-year period, and patients and staff had eventually become familiar with their sectors when it was decided that the sector limits should be different, in that the sector boundaries for somatic and psychiatric care were to be broken down. This is a sensible proposal in itself. However, for some hospitals it meant having to serve completely different sectors than they had previously. Gaustad Hospital, for example, had to take over sectoral responsibility for an area it had not held previously, whilst its old sector area was taken over by another institution. For patients who had been attached to the institution for a number of years, and who from all the relapses were used to coming here and getting their service from 'their' hospital with for example in-patient care, day care and after-care, it was obviously a severe factor of uncertainty to be turned away from this place and have to find a sense of belonging somewhere else. Although rules were issued for gentle transitional arrangements, it is not easy to accomplish this with shortage of space in institutions. There is no doubt that such administrative shake-ups cost lives, regardless of how good the rules established for gentle transitions are.

Another factor in recent times has been the shortage of space in Norwegian psychiatric hospitals. There have been severe restrictions on beds in psychiatric hospitals, as exemplified by the decline at Gaustad, from around 600 patients at the start of the 1970s to less than 200 patients at the end of the 1980s. It is the in-patient places on which there has been most pressure, and the worst and most difficult patients which the hospitals have difficulty coping with. The result has been that there are problems in very many Norwegian psychiatric institutions over transfers from open to closed wards, if the behaviour of the patients becomes too difficult or the danger of suicide dictates that they should be treated in a closed system.

Statutory provisions have now obliged the psychiatric hospitals to take in cases which are defined as in need of immediate assistance, including suicidal patients. The hospital is under a duty to assess such patients and also to admit them if it is considered necessary. It is quite clear that the chronic shortage of space in our psychiatric institutions means that the term immediate assistance can be stretched.

The development that has taken place in the direction of more and more beds being taken up by patients for immediate assistance means that it may be difficult to find space for patients who need more prolonged

treatment. These too often have to be admitted to emergency departments, and it is probably an unfavourable situation for many young
schizophrenics and long-term schizophrenics every time they suffer a
recurrence to be admitted to an emergency ward with all the activities, all
the turmoil, and the relatively short-term time perspectives there. No
sufficiently good models have been planned for more prolonged treatment of young schizophrenics and others in relapse, who may need more
long-term arrangements, in relation to psychotherapy, medicines and
social factors. Similar problems are being faced in neighbouring Nordic
countries.

With the restructuring that has taken place in both Norwegian and
western European psychiatry in recent years, there is reason to believe
that the long-term patients have been the losers. They are the ones who
have been victims of the revolving-door policy which today unfortunately
plays a key role in psychiatry. This policy hardly helps to reduce the
incidence of suicide.

What can be done?

Something has to be done. We probably cannot go back to the old, strict
security system. However, we have to devise better measures. It is
important that all staff are well informed about patients who are regarded
as potential suicides. It is also important that all patients who are
regarded as being at risk from suicide are admitted to hospitals and that
they are not met with rejection, being told that there is no room for them
here, or that the situation is very difficult today because of sick leave,
holidays, etc. The patients should be able to feel welcomed by the
institution where they are received, and they should be taken in at once if
the danger of suicide is judged to be great. It is important that attending
doctors give themselves time in the initial conversation with the patient
and it is also important for nurses and environmental staff to meet the
patient in a positive manner. A particular contact should be attached to
suicidal patients – contacts who in a discrete way can also pass onto staff
information on how the patient is developing. Ample time should be
given for the patient to settle down in the ward. One should be cautious
about sending the patient out in the early period without follow-up. One
should also generally wait longer before granting home leave to a patient
who is considered to be at risk from suicide. Contact should be made with
the family to arrange forms of supervision during the home leave. A
patient who feels isolated, overlooked and devoid of contact with staff

will be in greater danger than a patient who has good contact. The former will also display aggression towards the staff. There is a greater chance of this aggression being directed inwards, with the consequence of attempted suicide. Attempted suicide can also indirectly represent a protest against the attitude of staff, an aggressive act with an appeal for more care and attention.

The suicidal patient should be looked at from a longer time perspective than just the stay in the ward. It is often a long-term arrangement, where the after-care is particularly important, and contact later must be maintained over a long period – often years.

In my view significantly more effort should be made in psychiatric hospitals and clinic wards on the assessment of suicidal patients and making arrangements for them. Guidelines should be drawn up on how to act towards them. There should be a permanent reporting system from one shift to another, that is from day shift to afternoon shift to night shift. Reports should be kept and there should be ultimate control of the plans. It is also important for personnel to be familiarised with routines, for example in connection with meetings, which take up an increasing proportion of the working day in psychiatric hospitals. When staff meetings are taking place, it must always be ensured that sufficient staff are nevertheless present to supervise the patients. The opportunities for taking one's own life are greater during these periods when staff are occupied with meetings. In the future we shall without doubt work towards reducing the time spent on meetings and increasing the time spent with the patients. Far too large a proportion of time is taken up by staff meetings of various kinds and administrative meetings.

Education and training in the subject of suicidology

The level of knowledge of suicidology (the science of suicide) is still not sufficiently high in psychiatric institutions, either among doctors, psychologists, social workers, nurses or other environmental staff. The subject of suicidology has been a neglected area in Norway as in many other countries. The subject of suicidology must be given far greater emphasis in the teaching of medical specialists, psychologists and other occupational groups. As things stand now, only systematic teaching is given in the subject at the University of Oslo medical curriculum in the form of four hours of lectures, but the subject obviously forms part of psychiatry teaching and teaching in other subjects, for example internal medicine. However, the amount of instruction given is still too small.

Psychology students also receive little systematic instruction in this subject. However, increased teaching of students is not enough. The subject of suicidology must be taught continuously. In further and advanced training courses for doctors at universities, the subject of suicidology should be a subject which is repeated at fixed intervals. In psychiatric hospitals it is important that instruction in suicidology be given at least once every six months. There is always a significant turnover of staff in our institutions, and new staff must study the subject of suicidology. It is possible to plan such courses so that both doctors and nurses and health personnel can derive benefit from them, something which the author has experienced both in his own hospital and around the country.

If there has been a suicide at a hospital, it must be closely examined. It is important that the attending physician, psychologist and departmental staff discuss the case at staff meetings, preferably several, where any errors made are examined and where it is possible to learn so that another suicide on a later occasion can be prevented. As a rule it will also be an advantage for the suicide to be discussed with the patients, if they know about it. They may have questions to ask which can be answered without breaking the duty of confidentiality, and they also have a need to mourn which can be important to deal with.

Suicide probably cannot be completely prevented in a psychiatric institution. In an interesting book, *Suicide. Inside and Out* by Reynolds & Farberow (1977b) have attempted to shed light on the prospects. One of the authors (the sociologist Reynolds) arranged for himself to be admitted to a psychiatric hospital, supposedly after a suicide attempt, and presented symptoms of being at great risk of suicide. He went through all the procedures applicable to patients threatened by suicide, and was treated as though he was in the highest risk group. The researcher carried out the plan satisfactorily, and managed to live up to the symptoms that were expected of him. Nobody suspected that he was not an ordinary patient. He noted that there were a number of opportunities open to him to commit suicide during the time when he was categorised as a suicidal patient. He also made a number of interesting observations on mutual communication between patients and on their role patterns. It appears quite clearly that it is extremely important to build up the patient's self-esteem. Where this self-esteem is undermined, if this is done with severe restrictive measures, the consequence will probably be an increased danger of suicide.

12

Psychological factors in suicide and attempted suicide

In chapter 7, I discussed Emile Durkheim's theory on social integration and the sociological factors which predispose people to suicide and attempted suicide (Durkheim, 1952). He emphasised that even if suicide may apparently be the result of the personal characteristics and situation of the individual, in reality it is a consequence of the social conditions. It is the moral and psychological climate of society which determines the size of the suicide figures. His theories are just as relevant today as they were nearly a hundred years ago. They are based on the view that man is primarily a social being who lives and acts in a society. We shall not repeat his theories here, but mention that he is often quoted as having compared society to a fire – those who are too far away from the fire freeze to death, those who are too close to the fire are burnt. In the case of excessively strong community feeling, altruistic suicide occurs, and if societal feeling is too weak, egoistic suicide occurs. If the control of society over the individual is too strong, fatalistic suicide occurs, if it is too weak, anomic suicide occurs. Fatalistic suicide takes place when the power and control of the community over the individual become too great. An example of an altruistic and political suicide in recent times is that of the Czech Jan Pallach in 1968 when the Soviet forces marched into Prague.

Freud studied the problem of suicide a great deal, although he did not produce a complete overview of the problem. In the 1920s he formulated the theory of the *instinct of death – Thanatos –* the aim of which was to remove bonds and thus destroy.

Freud believed that the instinct of death existed side by side with the instincts of life – sexual forces in the broadest sense. Whilst instincts of life are creative, the instinct of death is a force which works continuously towards death and towards bringing the living creation back to the lifeless, inorganic condition from which it actually originated. Freud also believed that the instinct of death was charged with energy and had to be displaced, and came to the view that both instincts, Eros and Thanatos, are the source of mental energy. As aggression which is turned inwards, against the individual himself, is dangerous to the individual, it must be tackled in such a way as to cause the least harm possible. This can be done in one of two ways, either by eroticising the aggression, that is combining the aggression with libido, lust, or by directing the aggression outwards against others. Freud suggested that suicide was originally a death wish directed towards others. This wish is then directed against the self to kill an object which has been established there by identification with key persons in early childhood.

Today we consider the dynamics of attempted suicide and suicide to be relatively complex. The dynamics generally consists of a discharge of aggressive tendencies directed against the individual himself, but also against others. In most cases a cry for help is also involved, and in some cases a need for punishment, of oneself or of others. The chances of survival in suicide attempts vary from almost certain death to almost certain survival. In many cases it will be Fate that will decide.

We have become aware in recent times of what an important role the early childhood situation has for our personality development. The influences on us in our first few months and years of life in many ways decide how we meet the problems of life later on. An interaction takes place between mother, father and child, and also with other important people. It is during the first few years of life that the most important foundation is laid. The love, care and warmth which we encounter may decide our security later in life. The more rejection, coldness and indifference we encounter, the more difficult it will be for us to develop a harmonious personality structure.

In the very first phase, the mother will be decisively important. The mother will generally do her utmost to meet the needs of the child, but some mothers may face problems because of their own illness, their own personality features and their own background, for instance if they have themselves grown up in difficult circumstances. There may also be difficulties in the marriage which means that the mother is left alone to care for the children, and has 'nothing to spare'. It has become clear in recent times that early loss of one or both parents, through death, divorce or other circumstances, may be detrimental to the development of personality and may predispose to later mental disorder. This is particularly the case where the child has not had any adequate parent substitute. There is often a clear predominance among psychiatric patients of early parental deprivation. The earlier the divorce takes place, the more detrimental it is if the child does not receive good and lasting parental substitutes. A particularly high incidence of early parental deprivation is found in studies of criminal, alcohol and drug abusers and suicidal patients.

It is unlikely that divorce, or the threat of it, in itself has provoked later suicide or attempted suicide. It is more likely that an insecure childhood makes the child unsure about establishing lasting, good social relationships with other people and predisposes the child to lasting emotional and social instability and uncertainty, something which in turn can predispose an individual to the type of crisis that induces the attempted suicide. If such a person is to establish good and lasting bonds with another person, he will be at greater risk if the bond breaks. The increasing suicide rate among young people in recent times may reflect the increasing tendency towards the break-up of families.

Emotional crises which trigger suicide attempts or suicide are usually those which provoke insecurity, weaken the person's self-image or threaten loneliness and reduced function in life. Crises of this kind include the loss of close and secure relationships, the loss or threat of loss of marriage partners, fiancé(e)s or sexual partners, severe frustration at work or at school, such as losing one's job or failing in examinations, prosecution, serious physical disorders and mental disorders. In most scientific studies of those who attempt suicide, 'erotic' conflicts or 'marital' conflicts are specified as the most common triggering factor in the attempted suicide, ranging between 30 and 80% in women. In men the conflict tends to be of a type that has to do with work, ambitions or self-esteem. In younger women, erotic conflict situations are most common, accounting for up to 80%.

Recent research has shown that our coping mechanisms are decisive in how we deal with the crises of life. There appears to be a combination of two factors in those who attempt suicide or take their own lives. The life crises are more difficult, greater in number and more complicated than for people who do not undertake suicidal acts, and the coping mechanisms are often weaker in those who attempt suicide. In addition there is often a lack of support in the social network. If such support is lacking, crises became deeper and the coping mechanisms poorer. It is not just the amount of stress that predisposes to suicide, but to a great extent the way in which the stress is tackled. The better placed we are in a social network, with contacts with family, friends, clubs, congregation, etc., the better our prospects of withstanding our stress reactions and dealing with them in an adequate manner.

However, a social network does not arise by itself. To achieve a good social network and maintain it, effort on the part of the individual is often needed, with commitment to others and to tasks. All research shows that those who attempt suicide have a smaller social network than the population at large, and the rest of the population has a larger circle of friends and acquaintances around it. Those who attempt suicide are less often members of groups or organisations such as clubs and congregations, they have less access to a telephone, and they receive telephone calls and letters from others less often. Poor or little contact with members of the family is a more common phenomenon for those who commit or attempt suicide than for the average population. A great deal can therefore be achieved in suicide-prevention work by helping people towards a better social network.

The three As in suicidology

The three As are of key importance in suicidology. They will usually be found both in suicides that have been carried out and above all in suicide attempts.

Aggression

This is directed against the individual himself, but in reality also against another person. This other person is referred to in suicidology as 'the important other'. It is generally a very close person, marriage partner, child, parent, employer, doctor or other person giving treatment. The individual who attempts suicide has often felt frustrated by the person in question, who has not given enough time and affection, or who has disappointed him in one way or another. The aggression which is actually felt against the other person is directed against the 'slighted' self.

Appeal

Appeal is very much a key word in suicidology. Most suicide attempts represent an appeal, *a cry for help*. The appeal is directed towards another person, usually the same person that the aggression is directed against, and the cry of distress contains a plea to bother more about the person concerned, give more time and affection, or the person concerned signals that he is a person in distress and in need of help.

Ambivalence

There is irresolution in most suicide attempts. It is rare to find a suicide which could not have been avoided, where all precautions were taken to ensure that the outcome was fatal. It is usual to find a door ajar. There is someone who is expected and who has not come, a rope which is too weak or a dose of medicine which at the limit of that which could kill. Ambivalence is a key word in suicidology. The suicide attempt is often a form of 'gambling with life', or something which the Germans call *die Gottesgerichtsfunktion des Suizidalversuches*. This entails challenging Fate or God, as in a game or lottery, and accepting the solution given. This has been expressed as 'the ordeal character of the suicidal attempt'.

The suicide attempt is generally a warning from the person that something has gone wrong in his life. Suicide attempts may come 'like a bolt from the blue', particularly for the 'important other', at whom the appeal is aimed. In cases of this kind the suicide attempt may, however, if it is tackled correctly and does not simply become the object of surgical or medical treatment, become the starting-point for beneficial subsequent development. With the assistance of a doctor or psychotherapist, the problems can be made conscious, so that the patient can talk through his problems, possibly with the therapist alone in a three-way conversation which also brings the important other person into the picture. The 'air' can be cleared in this way. Any person giving treatment should feel that the appeal function in the suicide attempt can be seen as an appeal, including to the person giving treatment, to look into the patient's life situation in more detail, and see into his difficulties better and understand him better.

Warning

Suicide generally comes as a shock to relatives and those around the person. However, most have given hints or warnings of what is going to happen. Three out of four do so. The hints are often indirect, such as drawing up a will or saying that one is afraid of dying, but they can also be clearer suggestions. We have examined this situation earlier. Here we shall merely repeat that suicidal threats must be taken seriously. In my student days I learnt that those who talk about suicide do not commit suicide. Today we know that a person who reveals suicidal thoughts to another person is ten times more likely to take his own life than a person who does not express such thoughts. It is a widespread misconception that people who talk about suicide will not commit it.

13

Suicide and biochemistry

We have not yet reached the stage where biological factors can be brought into the picture to any great extent when the risk of suicide is to be assessed. But progress has been made in this area since the previous edition of this book was published. This research mostly dates from the 1980s. This short chapter is aimed at those with a special interest who want a brief introduction to what is new in this area. In the Nordic region it is Marie Åsberg and her group at the Karolinska Hospital in Stockholm, Sweden, in particular who have researched this topic.

Since the 1960s, measurements of the signal substances 5-HIAA (5-hydroxyindolacetic acid, the metabolite of serotonin) and HVA (homovanillinic acid of dopamine) and HMPG (or MPHG, 4-hydroxy-3-methoxyphenylglycol, the metabolite of noradrenaline) in spinal fluid have been made on depressed patients without any conclusions being reached on whether the occurrence of these substances was reduced or not.

As a result of improved analytical methods and consistent work with a strict selection of patients restricted to the form of depression known as melancholia, both Swedish and international research groups have been able to show that the content of 5-HIAA and HVA in the spinal fluid is reduced during depression.

It is obviously not possible to pronounce on this basis whether depression is due to disturbances to serotonin turnover, or dopamine or noradrenaline disturbances with respect to breakdown.

It has been shown that around a third of melancholically depressed patients have a low level of 5-HIAA in the spinal fluid, and that such a low level is found in a few healthy individuals. It is interesting that the healthy persons with a low 5-HIAA level more often than expected have relatives who have been depressed. This suggests a possibility that a low 5-HIAA level may be a marker of increased (possibly genetically caused) *vulnerability* to certain mental disorders. The disturbed serotonin turnover generally also appears to persist after the patients have become healthy, which could be expected if it was a vulnerability marker.

One-third of depressed patients also show signs of disturbed serotonin metabolism. Does this mean that they differ clinically from other depressed patients? The answer to this question is possibly yes.

There is now evidence that patients with a low 5-HIAA level react less well to traditional antidepressants. An even more surprising finding is that patients with a low 5-HIAA level appear to have a significantly greater tendency than other depressed patients to attempt suicide; their attempts at suicide are also serious ones. A follow-up study has shown that the death rate from suicide in those attempting suicide who have a low 5-HIAA level is ten times higher than in other patients who have attempted suicide. The increased suicidal tendency associated with a low 5-HIAA level in the spinal fluid was described for the first time in Sweden, but has since been confirmed in groups of patients in the USA, Great Britain, the Netherlands and Hungary. It is therefore one of the best replicated findings.

This does not mean that an answer has been found to the problem of assessing the risk of suicide. Obviously a realistic model of suicidal behaviour in particular involves social and psychological factors, but the biological factors do appear to play a part.

We know from animal experiments that serotonin turnover is significant for some aspects of aggressive behaviour. It is possible by inhibiting the synthesis of serotonin to transform tame domestic cats into raging wild animals or cause rats which are nursing their offspring to bite the young to death.

In order to assess the relationship between aggressiveness and the occurrence of 5-HIAA in the spinal fluid, experimental studies have been performed in man. A projective test in psychiatry is the Rorschach test, which provides various information on the subject's personality. 'Blind' Rorschach assessments have recently been performed in which it was found that there was agreement between the results of the Rorschach test and the occurrence of 5-HIAA in the spinal fluid of psychiatric patients. A low level of 5-HIAA occurred statistically significantly more often in individuals in whom the Rorschach test showed a higher level of aggressiveness and anxiety. In the USA a link between the number of open aggressive episodes in military personnel with various types of personality disorder and the level of 5-HIAA in the spinal fluid was described. It thus appears that the hypothesis of aggressiveness as a mediating variable between serotonin and suicide has gained some support.

The results that have emerged so far on serotonin metabolism suggest that 5-HIAA determinations in the spinal fluid are not suitable for routine use. However, they can form the starting-point for attempts to find other targets for the serotonin turnover which can be used on a larger scale.

From a review by Braverman & Pfeiffer (1985), the following are of particular interest.

The following are found in depressive disorders: reduced $5\text{-}HT_2$ in the frontal lobe (Stanley & Mann, 1984), reduced 5-HIAA in the spinal fluid (Ninan *et al.*, 1984; van Praag, 1983), reduced magnesium concentration, reduced serotonin in the spinal fluid (Banki *et al.*, 1984), reduced melatonin in the cerebrospinal fluid, reduced HVA in the cerebrospinal fluid (Ziporyn, 1983). All these findings correspond to the hypothesis that serotonin and catecholamine activity is reduced in groups of suicidal patients.

In other studies reduced MAO in platelets (Ziporyn, 1983) and reduced imipramine receptor binding in the frontal lobe (Stanley, Virgilio & Gershon, 1982) have been found. This data agrees with another feature found in suicidal patients: impulsiveness. Stress and biochemical indicators are also implicated: increased plasma cortisol, increased 17-OHCS (Krieger, 1970), reduced TSH response to TRH (Ziporyn, 1983) and reduced uric acid in the urine. These findings have been identified by some researchers as common findings in suicidal patients, but cannot yet be regarded as definitely scientifically verified. In one study (Pfeiffer & Bacchi, 1975), patients with a high blood histamine concentration tend to be depressed and have a raised copper concentration in the serum, whilst pyroluric patients are impulsive and have raised cryptopyrrole in the urine: both groups appear to have an increased risk of suicide.

Two types of profiles of biochemical imbalance appear to be found in potentially suicidal patients:

(1) *depressive profile*, with reduced serotonin metabolism and high histamine concentration,
(2) *impulsive profile*, with reduced serotonin receptors, reduced catechol breakdown and pyroluria.

In addition to the links we have identified here, a statistical link has been found between suicide and a number of different substances in the body.

Raised values of 17-hydroxycortisone in the urine has been found to coincide with suicide. Plasma cortisol levels of over 20 mcg % are found to coincide positively with risk of suicide. The same applies to a positive dexamethasone suppression test (DSI). A very low response of thyroid-stimulating hormone (TSH) after the effect of thyrotrophin-releasing hormone (TRH) is also predictive of suicide. If the ratio between the quantity of urine and noradrenaline-adrenaline is low, there is a risk of aggression turned inwards, such as suicide. If the ratio is high, there is the opposite risk of aggression directed outwards.

It is emphasised once again that the research results which have been obtained on suicide and biochemistry for the time being have little or no practical application, but it can be predicted that in the future they will represent a valuable supplement in the assessment of the danger of suicide.

14

The suicidal process

A concept which is used today – the suicidal process – indicates a development from suicidal thoughts to completed action. Suicide attempts and suicide can be seen as quantitatively differing expressions of a fundamental suicidal tendency. It is the development from this tendency and its manifestations to the actual act that we call the suicidal process. This may begin early in life. The basis is often laid in early childhood. The successful existence of an individual will depend on how the individual succeeds in achieving good and secure relationships, first in the family circle and later within society at large.

We are now aware, thanks to the work of Bowlby (1969), that early loss of one or both parents through death, divorce or other causes is detrimental to personality development and can predispose the individual to later mental disorders, such as those we have considered. We have also mentioned that a significant predominance of 'parental deprivation' is usually found among psychiatric patients. The long development starts there. A lasting emotional and social instability and uncertainty may form in the individual which in time can predispose him to the type of crisis that can trigger suicide attempts.

We have also examined crises which trigger suicidal acts. These may be erotic conflicts and marital conflicts, loss and threatened loss of close partners, physical illness, change of environment or social isolation.

The suicidal process begins at some point along the way through life, generally during puberty or later. The actual process may develop over the course of days, weeks, months or years. It is a consequence of conspiring factors and evolves in a person in interaction with those in his

135

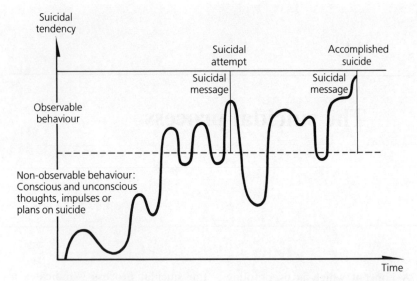

Figure 14.1. The suicidal process – development from suicidal thoughts to accomplished act. The figure shows how the person's involvement in the suicide problem changes over the course of time. Only small parts – above the broken line – become known to those closest to the person.

immediate circle. A curve of this suicidal process (Figure 14.1), given by way of a suggestion, has been produced following the 'care programme of the Swedish Board of Health and Welfare' (Swedish Board of Health and Welfare, Care Programme Committee 1983, p. 27).

When someone gets into an intolerable situation, from which that individual can see no way out, the thought comes of escaping the torment and misery, and of dying. There can also be positive effects in such suicidal behaviour, in that anxiety is alleviated through the discovery that an end can be put to the torment. Thoughts of suicide can also serve as symbolic acts. The individual imagines the sorrow and guilt feelings of relatives when they are told what has happened. Informing those close to them, someone with suicidal thoughts may also arouse sympathy and affection, and get those who are close to pay more attention to them.

The negative consequences are primarily the risk of early death or physical injury. Repeated suicidal acts can also become an escape mechanism from problems.

The person concerned often becomes increasingly engrossed in thoughts of suicide, asks himself whether life has any meaning, swings to and fro in his assessment and uses up a great deal of energy on the problem. Symptoms such as we have examined – depression, a feeling of hopelessness and loss of overview – tend to come during this development. The person concerned is said to have 'tunnel vision' or to be 'blinkered', unable to get a good all round picture of life. During the next period the person is often quite unstable. He regards the time and the situation as annoying, hopeless, and often seeks help from people around him. Minor difficulties become major ones, and he feels that disaster is looming.

Some suicidal acts occur after much deliberation and may be in line with the person's life-style. In others the act comes more spontaneously and without reflection, and happens in a state of chaos, anxiety, depression or under the influence of alcohol.

A period of suicidal wishes is often followed by a quieter period. When the person in question encounters fresh problems or suffers a bout of mental illness, the suicidal thoughts can crop up again. Constant reports of such thoughts, even if they appear half-hearted, can tell the world around that something is wrong.

The suicidal process can start at any age. It can begin in the teens, it may be chronic or it may be acute. If something happens which relieves the pressure, the suicidal process can enter a quiet phase, and almost remain dormant there. But in others the suicidal thoughts may be chronic companions through life. In the vast majority of cases the suicidal process does not develop further to suicide, and for some people the thoughts fade right into the background again.

It is said that suicidal messages and suicide attempts can be a great burden on the family. On the one hand it can help the family to establish contact with the person who is threatened, but on the other hand it may have the effect they become fed up with the person in question and simply keep their distance and retreat, because they find it a great strain. It induces anxiety in those around, and can cause them to give up. It is not unusual for the immediate family in one way or another to have understood that a suicide attempt or suicide is imminent but not be able to do anything more because over long periods, perhaps years, they have found the situation too much of a strain for themselves. Suicide can obviously be a severe blow for the family and cause wounds which never heal, but it can also lead to a form of clarification and relief.

The presuicidal syndrome

The Austrian suicide researcher Ringel (1953) described three phases which precede a suicide:

(1) *Narrowing and isolation* with loss of expansive forces, stagnation, passiveness and lack of ideas, lack of independence, clinging and perplexity. The scope for action is narrowed, the view of the world around becomes more and more one-sided. The narrowing of human contacts means that there is a tendency to avoid others and seek more and more isolation.

(2) *Aggression* of various kinds, primarily directed against oneself, and ultimately unsatisfactory discharge of aggression outwards in the form of accusatory suicide notes. The presuicidal syndrome sometimes includes a calm and serene attitude which can be misinterpreted as an improvement and may only become understandable afterwards.

(3) *Flight from reality*, with fantasies and daydreams, but also with dreams and fantasies about committing suicide. The process is completed with the suicidal act itself.

This process is developed in close interaction with other people who are close to the person concerned. Their understanding and support may be just as important as their hopelessness, abandonment and perhaps finally tacit sanctioning of the suicide. The suicide attempt is often the first sign that a suicidal process has begun, and serves as an alarm signal which may represent a definite turning-point in a person's life.

Others have tried to divide the presuicidal progression in different ways. Walther Pöldinger, a leading figure in suicidology, has attempted to divide the progression into three phases (Pöldinger, 1968).

(1) *The deliberation stage* is what he calls the first stage, where the individual considers suicide as a possible answer to his problems. The reason why suicide enters the individual's thoughts may be that there has been a suicide among friends and acquaintances, in the family or that the problem has been encountered in the press, in literature or in films.

(2) *The ambivalence stage* is where a struggle takes place between the self-building and self-destructive forces which are contained in everyone. In this phase suicidal threats emerge which are partly appeals or cries for help and act as a kind of safety valve. The internal battle between self-building and self-destructive urges is an expression of the ambivalence with which many who commit or attempt suicide struggle. An individual wishes on the one hand to live and on the other to die, but if he is to continue living, he wishes to live differently. It is important for those

around the person to listen to the signals the person gives during this phase.

(3) *The decisive stage* is the stage when the person in question takes a decision. A certain calm will often descend, which may appear striking to those around the person. Many people unfortunately draw the conclusion that the danger is now over, whereas in reality it is a lull before the storm. If the person in question has decided to carry on living, it will usually be possible on inquiry to discover what plans he has, the targets he is working towards or solutions he can see. Those who have decided on suicide will answer far more vaguely and evasively. At this stage those who will commit suicide often settle up, by paying off old debts, giving presents to friends or family or giving away jewellery they are fond of and which is of sentimental value to them.

The prototype of a person who commits suicide is an elderly man, single, separated, divorced or widowed, who lives in a rented room or lodgings, who has no job, has alcohol problems, is depressive and in addition has a physical disorder.

The prototype of a person who attempts suicide and survives the attempt is a younger unmarried woman in her twenties who is in an erotic conflict situation with the imminent break-up of a relationship, engagement or marriage, or with a break-up that has just happened.

A number of psychological test methods have been devised which are designed to be able to predict the degree of danger of suicide. They are partly 'rating scales' where the person concerned has to cross off boxes on a form, and partly more intricate rating scales where the person giving treatment or staff has to cross off a number of items of data. There appears to be agreement among specialists that at present there is no psychological test method which can predict with any degree of accuracy whether a person who is in a suicidal process will commit suicide. Ultimately it is the person giving treatment who must assess this on the basis of an in-depth knowledge of the patient and resources in the world around.

Performance of the attempted suicide

The suicide attempt will usually be carried out with more or less planning, and there will very often be a possibility of someone intervening. The act itself results in differing types of harm with varying probability of survival. We shall present an overview of this in Table 14.1, in line with the overview given by the Swedish Board of Health and Welfare (1983).

Overall picture of the suicidal process

In the report from the Swedish Board of Health and Welfare (1983), it is stated that an analysis of conscious suicidal tendency, suicidal message or suicide attempt is not sufficient to obtain an overall picture of the suicidal process. It is also necessary to study the first occurrence of the suicidal thoughts – when, where, how and why – and the subsequent development of these phenomena, including an analysis of the suicide attempt itself. The intention is to understand what situation or situations the patient cannot tolerate and what factors reduce or increase the risk of suicide. The following factors are among those which are of significance:

(1) The patient's personality, the difficulties he faces and how he responds to these, in particular situations which have formed the basis for the suicidal act or the symptom.
(2) The situation, difficulties and attitudes of other people close to the patient, particularly in connection with suicidal behaviour.
(3) The patient's experience of life and death – deaths, suicides or divorces in his childhood and later.
(4) The patient's view of the future – his own judgment of the risk of repeated suicidal acts, and his view of how long he is likely to live and how he will die.
(5) Occurrence of indirect self-destructive behaviour, such as abuse of alcohol and tablets, violence or threat of violence against another person, 'risk-taking behaviour', tendency to be accident-prone, and general lack of planning in conducting his life.

Table 14.1. *An overview of the performance of attempted suicide*

Probability	Of survival	Of someone intervening
None, or almost none	Shot into parts of body such as head or body. Jumping from a great height. Hanging. Toxic substances which are immediately fatal.	Lonely place with no access to telephone, such as in forest, at a remote place, in a barn, etc.
Low	Taking of large quantities of hypnotics, antidepressants or narcotics. Drowning attempts, poisoning with exhaust fumes or domestic gas. Suffocation, deep wounds on neck.	Alone, intervention of passers-by possible but not likely. Hotel room, alone at place of work in the evening. At home when no one is expected. Telephone can be found but is not used.
Moderate	Taking small or moderate quantities of hypnotics, antidepressants or narcotics. Large doses or combinations of different medicines. Other moderately toxic substances. Deep slash wounds requiring suturing of vessels or tendons with exception of a single wrist wound. Several deep wounds.	Alone and no certainty of immediate help, but reasonable chance of someone coming, e.g. of someone being expected. Telephone is available and can be used to summon help. The suicide attempt is hinted at beforehand.
High	Taking small or moderate quantities of tablets, benzodiazepines or neuroleptics. Slash wounds in wrist requiring extensive suturing, possibly of vessels and tendons.	Other person who can be expected to make contact is nearby, but outside visual range.
Very high	Taking non-toxic chemical substances such as baking powder, mouthwash, etc. Taking tablets, benzodiazepines or neuroleptics at slightly more than therapeutic dose. Slash wounds which do not need to be stitched.	Attempt made in presence of another person.

15

Assessment of the danger of suicide

This is one of the most difficult tasks in medicine and psychiatry. Every experienced doctor or nurse will have experienced suicide where they have assessed the danger of suicide as low and experienced the tragic consequences such an incorrect assessment can have. No one can be skilled enough in this assessment. However, it is possible to make oneself more skilled through experience and knowledge. A number of factors are of significance in deciding whether the patient is a suicide threat or not, and how great the threat is. Some overview has been obtained on this through practical experience and through scientific analysis.

An overview is presented below of the important factors, but the sequence indicated will not necessarily reflect the seriousness of the danger of suicide when the specified phenomena are present.

Important factors

Sex

Men are at a significantly greater risk of suicide than women.

Age

The danger of suicide these days appears to be fairly equal from the age of 20 upwards, but with a marked increase in the risk after reaching the age of 80. The risk is particularly high for the younger age groups if drug or alcohol abuse is known, and the greatest increase has occurred in the younger age groups.

Family situation

People who live alone or are isolated from their family are more at risk of suicide than those who live in a family. Unmarried people are more at risk of suicide than those who are married, and the same is true of those who are divorced, separated or widowed. People who live in bedsits, in a boarding-house or in a hostel are more at risk than those who live in a flat or house with a family. There is a particularly high risk if a constant downward curve has taken place in the family situation, where one bond after another has snapped and where the person concerned has a very poor and thin social network, perhaps only associating with others who are in similar social misery. The better the network that can be built up around the individual, the better the chance that individual will have of being able to prevent suicide.

Previous suicide attempts

Persons who have made suicide attempts previously are significantly more at risk of suicide than those who have not done so. Those who attempt suicide and do not succeed are in a far higher risk group for subsequent death from suicide. Most studies show a greater danger of suicide among those who have made a suicide attempt which almost led to death than among those who have made a relatively 'harmless' suicide attempt which appeared to be more demonstrative. However, the difference is so small that in some studies no such link has been found, and it should therefore be borne in mind that even apparently 'harmless' suicide attempts may be accompanied by more serious suicide attempts that prove fatal next time.

Of those who have attempted suicide, 10–15% will die from suicide in the long run. This means that the majority of those attempting suicide do not die from the attempt. The more suicide attempts, the greater the danger of the person in question dying by suicide. People for whom suicide attempts have almost become a way of tackling life's problems, and who are admitted time after time with poisoning, and who often put a strain on the health system, are a group which must be anticipated as having a high probability of finally succeeding in taking their own lives.

Psychiatric disorders

We have previously discussed in more detail the significance of psychiatric disorders. Persons with psychiatric disorders which have involved treatment are significantly more at risk from suicide than others. A particularly high risk of suicide exists in *depressive* conditions, either of a manic-melancholic nature (major affective disorders) or of a reactive nature. The danger of suicide is also increased in depressive neurosis. Alcohol and drug abuse significantly increase the danger of suicide. The danger of suicide is also generally increased in *psychotic* conditions, particularly in *reactive* and *schizophrenic psychoses*, but also in psychoses in organic brain disorders and in what are known as borderline states or borderline-psychotic cases. Significant personality disorders also entail an increased risk of suicide.

It is extremely important that those who have psychiatric disorders are treated for them, and it is not least important that those who have completed treatment in an institution continue to receive after-care. This after-care should last for years or even life in many cases. During phases where contact in treatment is poor, where therapists change or the therapist is on holiday without giving notice or has not arranged a substitute, the danger is particulary great. The period immediately after discharge, particularly the first week, is a very high-risk period. The more commitment a therapist can give his patient, the better the after-care arrangements that can be offered, and the better the network contact that can be set up, the lower the risk of suicide becomes.

Physical disorders

Particularly serious disorders that may have a fatal outcome or lead to disability increase the risk of suicide. Among such disorders, mention may be made of cancers, chronic illnesses of other types and disorders which involve a great deal of pain and discomfort. However, there need not be a direct link between the seriousness of the physical illness and the danger of suicide. Many people may feel seriously worried about illnesses which to the doctor are relatively innocuous. The deciding factor is often to what extent the patient himself views the illness as dangerous or threatening, or how annoying the condition is, or how great the pain is. Hypochondriac disorders are associated with an increased danger of suicide.

Communication of suicidal thoughts, suicidal threats

The danger of suicide is significantly higher in people who communicate suicidal thoughts and make suicidal threats than among people who do not do so. As many as 60–80% of those who commit suicide have communicated their intention to do so earlier, usually in the form of suggestions or hints. It must therefore be taken seriously when people talk about committing suicide.

Preparations for suicide

Preparations are obviously signs of an increased danger. Buying weapons, ammunition, ropes or toxic substances are serious signs, as are preparations for what will happen after death: drawing up a will, deciding on hymns to be sung at one's funeral, discussions on how property and business are to be administered, worries about the situation of those left behind.

Occurrence of suicide in the family

The occurrence of suicide in the close family increases the risk. Some disorders which are associated with an increased risk of suicide have a hereditary component, such as certain depressive mental disorders, alcoholism and schizophrenia. More recent research also suggests that suicide in itself may be hereditary, and that it is necessary to be very cautious if it is known that there are one or more cases of suicide in the family.

Broken home before the age of 15

People from homes which have broken up before they were 15 years of age have an increased risk of suicide compared with those from stable, complete homes with two parents and who grew up in an 'uneventful' situation.

Unemployment and financial difficulties

Periods of unemployment, pressing financial problems, threats of going into liquidation and bankruptcy increase the risk of suicide. The same is true of setbacks such as failing in examinations.

Serious hypochondriac symptoms

Constant complaining, whining and worrying about physical symptoms, with anxiety about having physical disorders, increase the danger of suicide. This applies for example to the conviction that one has a serious disorder, such as AIDS, cancer, etc.

Sleeplessness

Great worrying in connection with persistent sleeplessness increases the risk of suicide. An increasing degree of sleeplessness is therefore an increased risk factor.

Biological crises

The danger of suicide is increased during biological crisis periods such as puberty, pregnancy, periods of childbirth and breastfeeding, and in climacteric conditions, which all involve disturbances to the hormone production and system of balance in the body. The same crisis periods are often accompanied by mental problems.

Loss of or primary lack of human contact

Loss of people who signify security, and on whom one is dependent, leads to an increased danger of suicide. This applies, for example, to the death of people to whom an individual is close, conflicts with them, divorce or threatened divorce. Becoming a widow or widower is also a high-risk period.

Conditions which signify a feeling of shame and defeat

These include prosecution, arrest, court proceedings, imprisonment etc. Both a feeling of guilt and a feeling of shame in connection with acts that one has carried out and cannot accept and which have become known to others increase the risk of suicide.

The presuicidal syndrome

As discussed earlier this syndrome must also be taken into account. *Narrowing* and *isolation*, *aggression* and *flight from reality* are associated with the presuicidal syndrome and further increase the risk.

Occurrence of suicide among friends and acquaintances

It is necessary to be on one's guard if a suicide has taken place in the person's immediate circle, as for example among close friends or a colleague. The same is true in hospitals. If there has been a suicide in a hospital or in a ward, it is necessary to be on one's guard for the next one. Suicide is to some extent 'infectious'.

In conclusion, an overview of the assessment of suicide risk presented by the Programme of Care Committee of the *Swedish Board of Health and Welfare* (1983) is given in Table 15.1.

Assessment on the basis of conversation with the suicidal patient

It is the conversation with the suicidal patient and what is obtained from it, together with what is known about the patient from talks with the family, that is the most important tool for assessing the situation.

Most health-care workers, including doctors, are opposed to the idea of talking about suicidalness with the patient. It is a taboo subject in all of us, and we feel unsure about provoking the patient in an area like this. The way in which the psychiatric interview is performed may be of decisive importance in the assessment. The person giving treatment must try as far as possible through his conversation to understand the process that has led the patient to a suicidal career, in other words to understand the suicidal process. This process will obviously be impossible to understand except through a precise analysis of the how the patient's life and illness have developed. It is often necessary to make a more direct approach than is usual in most psychotherapy situations.

There may be a danger of not having the suicidalness assessed if one does not raise the problem as a therapist. If a depressed patient or a person who is otherwise in a suicidal risk group does not mention their suicidal problems, it will be necessary for the specialist to bring up the subject by asking direct questions. One should obviously not rush blindly into the problem as one of the first things to be assessed. It is necessary first to get to know the patient and gain an insight into his life. But an effort has to be made and interest shown in finding out to what extent the person in question has previously attempted suicide, made threats or harboured thoughts. If the patient has made such an attempt before, it is important to find out about the circumstances, his thoughts and how the situation progressed. One should also find out about the fantasies the patient has had about his suicide plans.

Table 15.1. *Assessment of suicide risk*

	High risk	Risk which is difficult to assess	Low or no risk
Statistical risk factors	Many risk factors, e.g. the elderly, divorced, those living alone, unemployed, depressed man with alcohol problems and previous attempts at suicide.	One or a few risk factors.	No risk factors.
Conscious suicidal tendency	Thought-through suicide plans and active method at lonely place in near future.	Vague suicide plans with evasive answers.	Depressed mood. Suicidal wishes are denied in a convincing manner.
Suicidal messages	Clear repeated messages on serious suicidal thoughts.	Suicidal message with mixture of joking, seriousness and manipulation. Those around clearly worried, but patient denies problems.	No, or individual, suicidal messages in especially troubled situations, possibly under slight influence of alcohol.
Suicide attempt	Previous well planned serious suicide attempts.	Previous less well planned suicide attempts by passive methods.	No previous suicide attempts.
Overall picture of suicidal process	Repeated serious episodes of suicidal thoughts, with worked-through suicide plans and suicide attempts.	Many previous suicide attempts through slashing or poisoning, under influence of alcohol in order to be given attention.	No previous suicide history.
Problems, resources, relationships	Sudden, definite loss, e.g. divorce or bankruptcy.	Repeated break in relationships with close fellow beings which are sometimes repaired, sometimes not, increased social problems.	Problems for which there appear to be good prospects of coping and solving little by little.

	High risk	Risk which is difficult to assess	Low or no risk
	Family and good friends have long since given up apart from a few with whom the person is in conflict.	Relationships with relatives with double message. From the beginning good relationships which begin to weaken over the years with problems.	Good relationships with relatives who have the will and ability to stand up and help.
	Previous admissions to psychiatric wards under strong protest without person concerned understanding meaning of stay, feels psychologically abused and persecuted.	Attitude towards ward staff fluctuates between open hostility and ingratiating behaviour.	Mutual respect and trust between patient and ward staff.
Physical illness	Fatal, painful, disabling illness, e.g. in genital organs. Diseases in hypochondriacs.	Less serious physical illness with symbolic meaning.	Physically healthy.
Mental disorders	Depressive psychosis, severe schizophrenia.	Brain damage, long-term asthenic depression or compulsive neurosis. Impulsive acting-out personality.	Mentally well.
Abuse	Severe alcohol and/or drug abuse in connection with social degradation.	Moderate or periodic alcohol abuse which causes depression, feelings of guilt and aggression during and after inebriation.	No abuse.

One should be aware during the talk that people who are threatened by suicide are often highly sensitive and can be easily made to feel rejected, and experiences of rejection can precede the suicide or attempt. One must be very cautious about confrontations and admonishments. One should not be forceful in the examination, but try to achieve empathy, create understanding, warmth and affection, and if possible develop a positive transfer relationship in this phase. The person talking should be secure in the situation and not allow himself to be provoked by any aggression, which often also accompanies the suicide problem.

The patient's attitude and behaviour during the talk may be of great significance. If there is a great deal of aggression directed inward, and if the patient, for example, has many thoughts about earlier losses and defeats he has suffered or fantasies about his own death, these will be factors supporting the view of the danger of suicide. The demonstration of hopelessness and fear of loss of control points in the same direction. If the patient discusses the consequences of suicide and how things will be later for those left behind him, these are obviously danger signals, as is emotional instability.

In relation to psychiatric patients such as schizophrenics who perhaps live in a marginal state outside, it is important to analyse how the patient experiences this phenomenon, and for depressives it is important to analyse what chances they see of getting back to their normal ego again. It is very important to assess the resource situation of the patient. This can partly be done by talking to patients and hearing what their relationship is like with, for example, their marriage or cohabiting partners, parents, children, and to what extent the person in question can expect help from them. If the relationship is a positive one and support and help can be counted on, this points in a positive direction.

The occurrence of the presuicidal syndrome obviously increases the danger of the person in question committing suicide. This syndrome has already been discussed. As mentioned there, the most important symptoms of the presuicidal syndrome are:

(1) Narrowing and isolation.
(2) Aggression.
(3) Flight from reality.

The therapist who is to assess the danger of suicide will always face many uncertain factors and will generally be in doubt as to how to act. If the danger of suicide is regarded as high, and a psychiatric disorder of a more serious nature is present at the same time, admission to hospital will be indicated in most cases.

Assessment on the basis of biological factors

The biological aspect of suicidalness was previously restricted to the assessment of the degree to which the patient was burdened by a manic-melancholic mental illness in the family, or physical disorders. The occurrence of such a 'major affective disorder' or a manic-melancholic disorder is a risk factor that is beyond doubt when it is considered that the risk of suicide in patients with such disorders is 15% over the course of their life. But we also know that groups with serious somatic disorders are at high risk of suicide. We have discussed this situation earlier in the book.

Modern biochemical research has made findings which emphasise the importance of including biology when assessing suicidalness. A lowered level of 5-hydroxyindolacetic acid (5-HIAA) and 3-methoxy-3-hydroxyphenylglycol (MHGP) in the cerebrospinal fluid appear to be indicators of a significantly increased risk of suicide among depressive patients. Although there is some way to go before such methods can be put to clinical use, the research in progress in this area indicates that the biological profile in future will have to form part of the assessment of the suicidal patient. The biochemical factors are discussed in chapter 13.

Assessments on the basis of socio-cultural factors

These have been examined in depth in the first part of the book, and apply to factors such as sex, age, marital status, etc. These factors must be seen in connection with the life situation the patient is living in, and also be assessed on the basis of traumatic events such as, for example divorce, death of the marital partner or a close friend, or conflicts with the family, which may have preceded the current situation. Such external factors will obviously increase the danger of suicide. The same is true of social isolation and the various types of psychiatric disorders we have examined so far.

The assessment also includes an appraisal of the resources around the patient – to what extent can an effort be anticipated, to what extent are there resourceful people around the patient and to what extent are these people willing to make an effort? It can often be important for the therapist in collaboration with the patient to make contact with potential resource people.

Assessment on the basis of sociological and psychopathological understanding models

These factors have also been discussed in depth in previous chapters of the book, to which reference should be made (e.g. chapters 7, 12). Psychiatric diagnosis in itself is only one factor which can be brought in, but the whole life-story and case history must be included as well. Previous attempts, suicidal thoughts, etc., always increase the risk.

Diagnostic systems used in psychiatry have changed at various intervals. At present ICD-9 (International Classification of Disorders, edition 9, WHO 1977) is used in Norway, but use is also made for research purposes of the American diagnostic system DSM-III and DSM-III-R (Diagnostic and Statistical Manuals, from the American Psychiatric Association, 1987). The use of these diagnostic systems in itself is unlikely to be decisive in our assessment, apart from what has been said earlier about psychiatric disorders in general.

Assessment on the basis of intrapsychic factors

We have also discussed these factors in earlier parts of the book. Aggression, appeal and ambivalence are involved here. A feeling of anger, hatred or hostility towards people to whom one is close and on whom one is dependent for love and affection can easily be directed against oneself and lead to self-destruction. If one feels let down by one's marital partner, parent, child and not least by the doctor or therapist, the aggression may instead be directed against oneself. Affection and hatred are closely linked.

When someone one is close to dies, a wish to be re-united with the deceased can also be experienced, and in the case of pathological mourning, suicide may occur.

In intolerable situations in life, such as for example, chronic and painful disorders, torture, the fantasy of the possibility of suicide can represent confirmation that the ego still has autonomy and is capable of influencing the situation.

Many who attempt suicide have what is referred to as a 'dichotomic' way of thinking, That is thinking in diametric opposites, where the attitude is characterised by the concepts of life and death being in stark contrast to one another and clear alternatives to one another. This way of thinking is also assumed to increase the risk of suicide.

The presuicidal syndrome has been discussed in detail in chapter 14.

Finally the manner in which the suicide attempt was made is assessed if the person concerned survived, that is the chance was small or great of the person being saved. But as we saw earlier, the risk of suicide is not greatly increased because it was a dramatic suicide attempt.

16

Popular misconceptions about suicide

People who talk about suicide will not commit suicide
As mentioned earlier, this is incorrect. If people talk about suicide, it must be taken seriously.

Nothing can be done about those who make serious attempts at suicide – they will commit suicide sooner or later
This is a claim that is false, since only 10–15% of those who have made serious attempts at suicide die later from accomplished suicide.

Those who are under treatment by a doctor, for example a psychiatrist, do not commit suicide
Psychiatric patients have a higher incidence of suicide than others, as we have just seen.

Suicide comes without warning
This is an incorrect claim. In most cases of suicide, the patient has given direct or indirect warnings beforehand.

It is not difficult to understand why he committed suicide, life was very difficult for him
There is always a reason for committing suicide, but if it is looked at in greater depth, the background will always be more complex and difficult to review, and very many people get into similar or greater difficulties without committing suicide.

Suicide affects a certain social group in particular
As already discussed, suicide affects the various social groups fairly equally, and is quite 'democratic', although it is the highest and lowest social groups which seem to be at greatest risk.

Good living conditions militate against suicide
This does not appear to be correct. The suicide rate is high in the modern welfare state, and has risen as the economy and welfare have been improved.

Suicide is hereditary
This does not hold water. There may be an accumulation in some families of certain disorders which are accompanied by suicide, such as manic-depressive psychosis or alcoholism. Suicidal behaviour to a certain extent can also be learnt from experience during childhood, but the behaviour as such is not inherited biologically.

It is easy to find the motive for suicide
As a rule there is not just one motive. Each 'cause' found is usually preceded by another 'cause'. A long series of causes with suicide as the final solution is most common.

Suicide is an insane act
This can be discussed, but as we have seen, relatively few suicides are triggered in insanity.

17

Treatment

Treatment outside of hospital – treatment in the primary health service and social services

Some cases of attempted suicide are without doubt so innocuous that neither patients nor relatives consult a doctor. Anyone who has attempted suicide should undergo medical treatment, even if the attempt was not so serious that the patient's physical condition has made it necessary to call a doctor. The suicide attempt in itself is a warning that something has gone seriously wrong in the patient's life. The relatives and the patient should discuss the problem with the doctor or other representative of the health service. The primary health service will thus be the first organisation to enter the picture. Some patients will also come into contact with the social services, which are also responsible for people in distress, not least for groups who are high-risk groups from the point of view of suicide, such as the elderly, homeless, problem families and drug and alcohol abusers.

Important tasks for the primary health service and the social services are to identify suspected or manifest mental diseases, such as, for example, depression of the melancholia type, for treatment in hospital. But the primary doctor will often be of great help to the patient and family. In some cases these are problems the doctor can discuss directly with the family, who can jointly reach an arrangement in an acute situation. The attempt may perhaps be an expression of the lack of a solution to a long-lasting and serious conflict situation where the parties involved need help from outsiders and from specialists. Or the attempted suicide may be one of many expressions of a more serious mental

156

disorder, a persistent neurosis or psychosis, an alcohol or drug problem, which can be treated. The primary health service can then ensure that the patient is examined by a psychiatrist or psychologist, or is admitted to a psychiatric clinic or hospital. The patient's own consent should preferably be obtained before he is admitted, but if it is a psychosis, a serious mental disorder, it may be necessary for the immediate family to request that the patient be admitted against the patient's own wishes.

The primary health service and social services may give significant help in acute crisis situations, in what is known as crisis intervention, which can take place by telephone, through home visits or through visits to a surgery. It is often important to be available and to be available *quickly*. The following factors are involved:

(1) Ensuring contact and attempting to create a compassionate relationship in the difficult and confusing circumstances that surround the person who has attempted suicide or the person who is in danger of suicide.
(2) Understanding the real and symbolic importance of the situation to the patient, and if possible predicting the risk of suicidal acts.
(3) Treating both the patient and his anxiety and the anxiety of those around him in connection with the situation.
(4) Focusing the conversation on the problem which is more relevant.
(5) Commenting on the patient's problems and also on the resources of the patient and those around him.
(6) Finally expressing conclusions as to what can be offered to the patient outside of an institution or whether admission is necessary.

The home environment is obviously particularly important. Are there resources available there or is the environment stretched and the resources exhausted? Does the doctor or primary health service staff have the skills, time, opportunity and commitment to treat the patient outside of an institution?

An assessment of these factors, and of the psychopathology in individual cases, will decide to what extent the primary health service itself must continue the treatment, which will then involve contact over a period of time, refer the task to a specialist in psychiatry, a psychiatric outpatients' clinic or have the patient admitted to hospital.

It is very important for the primary health service to plan for the correct situation for further treatment if this is considered necessary. Here the opportunities within the relevant sector must be assessed. Which hospital or which ward has shown itself most suitable for the assessment of suicidal patients, where does this patient fit in best? Motivation for admission by the patient is important, and time often has to be taken over this. It will generally be an advantage if the admission can be made by agreement with the patient, and in Norway in accordance with Section 4 of the Mental Health Service Act. Similar mental health laws are found in other western countries. If there is suspicion of psychosis, or there is a definite psychosis, admission under Sections 3 or 5 of the Mental Health Act will be relevant. It may be an advantage for the patient concerned to be able to see the ward where admission has been recommended. It may also be an advantage for the patient to come to the admitting institution for a pre-care talk, if time allows. Overall it is important to build up security around the patient, give care and support and be helpful, albeit in a discrete way, with motivation. If it is not definite that full-time treatment is indicated, day-hospital treatment may be considered, perhaps merely out-patient treatment in the form of an after-care arrangement.

Something that is very important in the primary health service is that the patient should not be rejected or gain the impression that he is a nuisance. I well remember from my own practical experience a patient, a student, who over a long period had had problems in his life which had resulted in depression that was so serious that he could no longer cope with his studies. However, he had a deep distrust of psychiatry, and could not stand the idea of undergoing psychiatric treatment. However, the situation finally became so hopeless and deadlocked for him that he plucked up courage, and one fine day he came to the psychiatric outpatients' clinic in his area. He had not, however, phoned beforehand, nor did he have any letter of referral with him. When he went to reception he was met with the comment that no one had time to deal with him there, because it was such a hectic day, and he did not have the proper papers with him. Being the modest man he was, he accepted this, but felt so frustrated because of the great effort he had made to consult a psychiatrist that he threw himself off the nearest bridge over a motorway. He broke his back. As a result he was admitted to the surgical ward, where he was detained for a long period. He was then transferred as a day-patient to the psychiatric ward with depression which was deep and required long-term treatment with both medication and psychotherapy.

The rejection he encountered in the out-patients' clinic was without doubt the straw that broke the camel's back. A therapeutic situation could probably have been achieved by giving up a few minutes to talk to him and giving him another appointment within the next few days. Many mistakes of this type are made daily. It is easy to overlook how important it can be to get to know the patient, listen to his complaints and try to arrange a consultation later on. An invitation to keep in touch by telephone may also be a good temporary aid which should be used more.

Mention was made earlier of the unfortunate aspects of the current restructuring of psychiatry with the establishment of new sectors, where patients become cannonballs fired from one institution to another, and may be rejected wherever they turn, or in any case are rejected in the sense that attempts are made to get the patient admitted elsewhere. Patients at risk of suicide are in need of continuity of care and concern, understanding and friendship.

Admission to hospital

As it is not within the scope of this book to discuss mental health laws throughout the western world, the Norwegian mental health laws have been used as an example to illustrate procedures that do take place.

The vast majority of people who have attempted suicide are probably admitted to hospital, to medical, surgical or other wards, depending on the nature of the attempt. We shall not look at the somatic methods of treatment for attempted suicide. They must come first in all cases. However, somatic treatment is never sufficient. When the patient has recovered after the suicide attempt, an effort must be made to shed light on his circumstances and where appropriate have him assessed psychiatrically. *A patient who has made a suicide attempt ought to have a right to psychiatric examination and treatment.* Often, however, neither the patient nor his family want a psychiatrist to be involved. It is then necessary to take time to motivate the patient or his family. It is primarily the doctors in the somatic wards who have responsibility for this. The internal medicine specialist or surgeon is not only responsible for the local intervention made, but also for the total patient, including the patient's circumstances. The doctor must therefore analyse the patient's circumstances, possibly in conjunction with staff such as, for example, psychiatrists, psychologists, social workers. If the patient is immediately sent back to the situation, little has actually been achieved. The patient himself will usually be keen to be discharged as soon as he has recovered, as for example after poisoning. This is an escape situation, exactly like the suicide attempt. The patient escapes from his problems, this time from having his problems addressed in hospital. It is important for attending staff in the hospital dealing with internal medicine, not to give in immediately to the patient's wish to be discharged, even though it might be useful to have a bed free for emergencies. One should take time to persuade the patient to allow himself to undergo further examination, and try to find out the reasons for the suicide attempt. The patient should only be discharged without the actual causes having been clarified as an emergency way-out. There is no doubt that in Norwegian hospitals patients are discharged far too quickly, and often without preparation. This is probably one of the most serious mistakes made in the treating institutions. However, we must not blame this entirely on surgeons and internal medicine specialists. Psychiatrists are not the most willing to have patients transferred to them if the somatic ward wants them to do so.

The period following a suicide attempt is a very good starting-point for reviewing and addressing the patient's life situation. The family is usually very committed to the problem at this time. They are at their most motivated for understanding and perhaps even helping. They are aware that when such a dramatic situation has arisen, there must be a serious underlying reason. People close to the patient should therefore be involved in the therapeutic situation. The suicide attempt should be seen as an appeal to the doctor to examine the person's life situation more thoroughly. There is no doubt that there is a massive disparity in Norway between the technical apparatus which is employed to save the patient's life and the apparatus employed to understand his mental background, help him with his problems and arrange circumstances better, so that a repetition can be prevented. The disparity is even greater with regard to the often inadequate help the patient receives when he tries himself out in society again. Immediate discharge from the medical ward after the patient's life has been saved is very regrettable, but unfortunately is all too common. The patient returns to the same life situation again, and is in great danger of making another attempt at suicide, possibly with a worse outcome. It is an advantage if a psychiatric consultant is attached to somatic wards. This is being done in an increasing number of places.

If there is doubt at the hospital as to whether the patient has a serious mental disorder, and if the suicide attempt may be a symptom of such a disorder, there is justification for admitting the patient against his own will under Section 3 of the Norwegian Mental Health Service Act. The admission in such cases should take place in the psychiatric department of the hospital or in a psychiatric hospital. The danger to his own life also means that the patient can be admitted under the immediate assistance provisions, including in the situation where the patient is not in an institution. If there is a convincing psychotic illness in the person who has attempted suicide, he can be transferred to a psychiatric institution under Section 5 of the Mental Health Care Act. In most cases, however, an attempt will be made to motivate the patient for such a transfer, so that the admission can be made under Section 4 of the Mental Health Care Act. Under both Section 3 and Section 5, the admission must be made at the request of the patient's next of kin, namely the husband or wife, if there is no major conflict, parents, children, brothers and sisters and grandparents. If there are no such persons, or they do not have a close relationship with the person in question, the request must be made by the health authority, social services office or police. In cases of compulsory admission, the patient must be advised of his right of appeal against the admission to the committee at the hospital. This committee is made up of four people, one of whom is a lawyer with the qualifications of a judge and one a doctor.

The fact cannot be concealed that it is difficult to get patients into psychiatric institutions in Norway. The number of places has been sharply reduced, probably further than is justified. In particular a shortage of secure places has arisen. It will therefore be found that questions are asked in psychiatric hospitals about the degree of suicidalness and the need for admission. However, a strong suspicion of suicidalness provides an entrance ticket to the hospital as an emergency. The hospital is not necessarily obliged to admit the patient for immediate assistance, but is obliged to assess the application and examine the patient, and where appropriate offer an alternative. We have previously discussed the unfortunate consequences of the constant changes of sector boundaries we have experienced, where patients who have previously been admitted to a hospital or a particular ward may perhaps on re-admission end up somewhere completely different. It takes time to establish contact and security.

Methods of treatment

A patient who is at risk of suicide or has made a suicide attempt needs to be cared for and watched over by staff. A patient at risk of suicide used to be put to bed, had to give up the possessions with which suicide could be carried out and was subjected to quite intensive supervision, usually in a secure ward. Nowadays such steps are avoided wherever possible. A discrete and considerate form of 'supervision' can be established by attaching a particular nurse to the patient or putting the patient in a small group which has permanent supervision from and contact with a nurse or a group of nurses. This person is referred to as a *contact*. However, there are constant changes of staff in hospitals who work on a roster, and it is also important to try outside of daytime, during the afternoon shift and the night shift, to establish a special relationship with the patient, so that he does not feel alone and deserted and left to his own thoughts. A balance must be struck between control and human contact. The patient must understand, and not least feel, that one wishes to get closer to him on the *human level*, and that the control system is not the primary aspect. It is only meant as a transitional arrangement in the most critical phase.

In the most acute phase it may be advantageous to have a special waiting-room or a small closed ward. If the ward is an open one, the manning situation must be particularly good – better than if it was a closed ward. There must be ample opportunity to consider the individual patient. Control of the patient must include ensuring that he is not allowed to store medicines which can be used for a suicide attempt, or that he is not able to open windows where he can jump from a great height.

One should be very cautious about home leave in the initial period following the suicide attempt. Experience from psychiatric hospitals shows that a substantial proportion of the suicides committed by in-patients are made during periods of home leave. Both doctors and nurses should therefore discuss home leave for a potentially suicidal patient in great depth. Contact must be made with the family, and if a patient is allowed out on home leave it must be agreed that a particular member of the family is responsible for supervising the patient. The patient should of course not be handed effective suicide weapons. It is important for the patient not to be exposed to unnecessary temptations during the most difficult phase.

The best prevention of suicide in the ward is an alert, well-trained, understanding staff who co-operate well with each other and with the patient. The better and the closer the relationship the patient has with the staff in the ward, the greater the chance of his informing the staff of his plans in one way or another. The greater the attitude of protest he adopts towards the hospital and staff, the worse the contact relationship is, the greater the chance that he will attempt suicide, and also omit to talk about his intentions. It is important to *stimulate the patient's self-esteem*. Patients at risk of suicide often have very low self-esteem, which one must try in various ways to raise and reinforce.

It is important for the patient not to be strictly controlled for too long. The easiest and safest thing for those responsible will obviously be to leave the patient for a long time in a closed ward under particularly close supervision. However, this may impose a strain on the patient. This may in itself provoke a fresh attempt at suicide, possibly proving fatal. It is better to give the patient gradually increased freedom, and progressively let him join in as many activities as possible in the hospital. It is not possible to establish general guidelines on who is to loosen the control. A guiding principle must be for the staff in the ward, including doctors, *to discuss the steps which are gradually taken, and for all who are concerned with the patient to be informed about it.*

Of other arrangements for treatment, mention must be made of occupational therapy and activities which will always be an important part of the treatment, and which should be started as early as possible, depending on the patient's situation. Other treatment arrangements include the contribution of the physiotherapist. It is important for the patient to be involved in physical activity. Gymnastics, athletics, dancing, music and riding will be beneficial. However, we shall not discuss these treatment activities in detail here.

Patients who have attempted suicide often have a tendency to project guilt onto the staff, to blame them for their misfortunes, and this in turn can lead to a negative feedback situation on the part of the staff. It is important to address these reactions in staff. It can be said that systematic work on feedback in the staff group is important. An active environmental therapy programme is an advantage, but only provided it serves to increase the patient's self-esteem by coping with new tasks. But the programme must also give the patient time and opportunity to address his problems. New problems constantly arise for the suicidal patient, for example with relatives, fellow patients and staff members, so it is important that the patient should be given the opportunity to communicate and discuss any problems with therapists or members of staff throughout his treatment. It is important to increase the staff's knowledge of the problems that can arise in the ward in connection with, for example the projection of guilt. It is of key importance that the atmosphere in the ward should be characterised by continuity, predictability, security and good communication. A combination of drug therapy and psychotherapy appears to be important.

Because many suicides take place in circumstances which entail separation, such as, for example, hospital admission, transfer to other wards or institutions, discharge, free exit or home leave or change of therapist, it will be necessary to discuss these situations in depth in the team. Rejecting and offending the patient must be avoided at all costs.

If a suicide occurs in the ward, it is very important for it to be thoroughly discussed. Post-mortem meetings with the doctors and staff can also serve to clarify the sequence of events in suicide, and analyse what has gone both right and wrong in the treatment. The meetings are often too superficial for the objective of a 'psychological post-mortem' to be achieved. However, they are necessary, because many of the staff, including the therapist, usually have a feeling of guilt and expect guilt to be projected onto themselves, which has also been done by other members of the team and not least the family. It may also be necessary to involve other patients in such meetings if they know about the suicide. A thorough discussion of a suicide in a hospital should be one of the essential routines and *never omitted*. There should be a special arrangement for those left behind by the person who has committed suicide.

Psychotherapy

The principles for the treatment of a person who has attempted suicide depend entirely on the underlying disorder. An important factor for the arrangement of psychotherapy is obviously correct diagnosis. It can be particularly important to assess the diagnoses of depression and character disorder, the latter as a borderline or narcissistic personality disorder. After the diagnosis has been established, it is necessary to plan and organise the psychotherapy. According to psychodynamic guidelines, it is important to promote the psychodynamic understanding, therapeutic attitude and therapeutic technique. In order to promote psychodynamics, it may often be necessary to have some preparatory talks with the patient and important persons within the family.

It is reasonable to base the individual psychotherapy following the attempted suicide on the dramatic action which has preceded it. It is essential for the therapist to achieve a good human relationship with the patient. He does this by listening and by allowing the patient to talk about his problems, but also by adopting an understanding and supportive attitude and exhibiting sympathy for the patient. It may emerge during treatment that the patient has been in conflict over a long period with one or more people, usually husband or wife, partner, fiancé(e) or steady girlfriend/boyfriend, parents, brothers, sisters or children. The conflict has generally not been discussed with the person or persons concerned. It is important for the patient in conversation to be made to address the background to the problems with someone who is neutral in the situation. The patient can gradually work out more positive ways of resolving conflicts, as he gets to know himself and his situation better. The attempted suicide often itself expresses an attempt to bring about discussion with a concerned person in order to be allowed to talk about the hopelessness or aggression, or to attract the attention of the other person concerned and make this person show more consideration. Very often it is also this person who has had to 'carry the can' in the attempted suicide, go and see a doctor, get the patient to hospital, warn the employer or ensure that the patient's work duties are covered. After the relevant problem has been clarified, it may be appropriate to work further on the driving forces which make the patient escape from his problems in the form of an attempted suicide instead of dealing with the problems to find a real solution in other ways. Threads leading back to a corresponding situation where the patient has chosen a flight solution rather than a real solution can often be found.

If the therapy goes further, it becomes *insight-oriented* therapy, where an attempt is made to draw the threads back to find the background to the patient's pattern of behaviour. Circumstances in the childhood home often have to be elucidated. The basis of the personality disorder which has predisposed the person to attempted suicide usually goes back to an early age. Where the patient's 'ego strength' is good, it may be appropriate to make him see some of the dynamic forces acting in him, and also to see the background to these. If the patient's ego strength is less good, and it often is, or if the circumstances otherwise are unfavourable, the therapist will merely clarify the current situation. In such cases a more *support-oriented* therapy can be organised.

During talks with the patient it is important always to be realistic and not promise more than can be offered. It is also important to take time to help, and not proceed too quickly with confrontations and deeper analysis. It must become clear to the patient through the therapy that it is the patient who must take responsibility for his life, and that the therapist can only help him along the way. Patients with suicidal problems often have significant aggression within them, aggression which is also directed against the therapist if he becomes involved in a deeper therapy situation. The patient may also provoke narcissistic forces which might exist in the therapist, and since every suicidal patient has usually been extremely sensitive towards narcissism, it may be the start of 'attacks' and difficulties in the therapy. It is, however, important for the therapist to be able to act consistently, calmly and predictably, and to guide the patient through this difficult phase, and preferably also continue with the therapy after discharge through after-care or out-patient treatment, perhaps over a long period.

Advice

It is important to offer the individual patient personally formulated assistance, in such a way that it does not lead to a positive reinforcement of depression or suicidal behaviour. Behaviour should neither be rewarded nor punished. An attempt must be made either to support the patient or to prepare him for constructive solutions.

An attempt should also be made to teach the patient different ways of controlling his anxiety by learning about the anxiety-provoking stimuli which can either be avoided or may be met with better understanding.

Co-operation with the family and ward staff is important. It is important to support the patient's self-esteem.

Must the patient be confronted with reality?

The patient is often unwilling to talk about his suicide attempt. In most cases the suicide attempt must not be allowed to appear as something mystical or uncontrollable – something which just happened – but the problems should be discussed and things that can be done to change the life situation should be looked at.

Caution must be exercised in the first phase. Suicidal behaviour is a consequence of the patient somehow having failed under the stresses of life. This should not be faced too clearly at first. Emphasis should be put on positive resources and identifying them in the individual.

The problems of aggression should be addressed in most cases. It may be favourable for the patient to gain an understanding of the fact that problems of aggression are involved.

Attempts should also be made to touch on family dynamics, and the family should be drawn into the picture to some extent, as we shall now see.

Family therapy

It will be desirable in both insight-oriented and support-oriented individual psychotherapy to talk to the family, and in particular with the person or persons the suicide attempt is directed against. The aim of this is to draw the family into the treatment, since patients mostly live in a family setting and it is in this setting that the suicide attempt has been triggered. The attitudes of family members towards one another and their way of talking to one another, may be of decisive importance to what happens afterwards. In such family therapy the patient talks to his closest family in the company of the therapist, who acts as a neutral and understanding third party. Much that has never previously been mentioned can be discussed. The patient may gradually become clear as to where he stands. Severe emotional discharges may sometimes happen, in the form of crying or anger. But this can have a purifying effect like a thunderstorm after sultry summer weather. The parties may perhaps gradually find a way out of their problems and come up with more tenable guidelines for the future. However, it may also become clear that they are in hopeless opposition to each other, and that the problems are virtually unsolvable. The best way out may perhaps be to sever the connection.

A scheme of treatment like this requires strong commitment on the part of the therapist in terms of both emotion and time. There is no doubt that the prospects are better if family therapy can be conducted in addition to individual psychotherapy. A suicide attempt will often lead to changes in the patient's relationship with those close to him or a larger group. It is important for these close people to be brought into the picture while treatment is still in progress. The aim of family therapy is to achieve greater understanding of the systems of communication in a family and to be able to change them. The suicidal patient has often become *the identified patient* in the family. Family therapy does not necessarily have to be conducted in an institution.

Group therapy

This form of therapy is particularly relevant in hospitals, and often forms an element in the general range of treatment offered. It is a form of treatment in which several patients participate, usually along with several therapists, and in which interpersonal problems are often discussed. Group therapy is conducted to a certain extent in the psychiatric institutions. There are no guidelines for what type of group a suicidal patient is to be placed in, and this will depend on whether the person concerned acts at the neurotic or psychotic level, and how strong the patient's ego is. There is experience in other countries of groups consisting solely of suicidal patients. The 'entrance ticket' for such groups is the situation of having been 'face to face with death'. It is a common finding, as for example in the USA, that there needs to be two therapists in such groups, because so much aggression emerges and one therapist alone finds it difficult to cope with it all.

Environmental therapy

Psychotherapy, individually, in groups and in families, will be cornerstones in the treatment of patients at risk of suicide in hospitals. However, there will also be *environmental* therapy. In recent years many people have come to the view that the environment in psychiatric institutions in itself is of decisive importance to the treatment. In a small community which a hospital ward can become, both doctors and treating staff in general can learn a great deal about the personality features and attitudes of the individual patient. The same attitudes which cause him difficulties in the small community of the hospital ward may perhaps also contribute towards the development of the suicide attempt or mental illness. We have nowadays become aware that environmental therapy may be strongly influenced by the patient's condition. In active wards that use confrontational therapy, it will be chiefly those patients referred to as the ego-strong and the resource-strong who will benefit from the treatment regime, and the ego-weak and resource-weak who will tend to be the losers. One must therefore be cautious about not only developing *active* environmental therapy wards, but also developing wards that work according to less ambitious principles in this respect but which can emphasise care, warmth and ego support for the weak. It is precisely this warm and care-oriented environment which those who attempt suicide often need, and it is ego support, encouragement and emphasis of positive resources that can often be the most important aspects for good treatment of the person who has attempted suicide.

Drug therapy

Drug therapy after attempted suicide must follow the same guidelines as medication in general. In mental illness the antipsychotic drugs, known as neuroleptics, will be given in the usual doses for the type of psychiatric disorder the patient concerned is suffering from. Melancholia and deep depression occupy a key position because many suicidal patients have this type of disorder, and patients with this type of disorder are also a high-risk group. At the same time it is specifically this group of psychiatric patients in whom the best results are achieved in treatment with medicines. Antidepressant medication given in correct doses can be the best suicide-preventing measure here. Melancholia can occur in many forms, and need not necessarily present only depressive symptoms. It is often possible to successfully help patients with what are known as *masked depressions*, which often have physically dominated ailments, with antidepressant medication. There is no doubt that the treatment of what are known as major affective disorders, which include melancholia, has not been sufficiently developed. The medication is often low, and half-treated melancholic conditions can predispose the patient to suicide.

A great deal can probably be achieved by doctors being trained in the drug treatment of depression. It is important for the treatment to be started early, and it is important for the dose to be sufficiently high. The maximum dose of tricyclic antidepressants which may be given in practice will usually be 150 mg, but 90 mg now appears to be an adequate maximum dose in general practice for the drug mianserin. There are still doctors who prescribe far lower doses, doses which are ineffective. If an antidepressant drug does not achieve anything, there is justification for trying another. However, it takes three to four weeks before the antidepressants work, and this can be a long time to wait for a patient who is suffering from severe depression. It is also important for doctors to choose drugs of low toxicity. Unfortunately, the tricyclic antidepressants are generally of high toxicity, but the more recent tetracyclics and monocyclics have a low degree of toxicity. It is clear that this is a great advantage specifically in relation to patients at risk of suicide, as these are usually depressive patients.

In cases where antidepressant medication is not successful, electroconvulsive therapy (ECT) may be the best treatment. In Norway there is a relative reluctance to give this treatment. Whilst around 10% of newly admitted patients in Denmark are given ECT, only 4% receive it in Sweden and just 2% in Norway. It is possible that lives could have been saved by electroconvulsive therapy started at the right time.

There has been a great deal of campaigning against electroconvulsive therapy from anti-psychiatry groups, and it is likely that doctors have become more reserved about the treatment for this reason and that this may have cost lives.

Today we have drugs for preventing manic-melancholic psychosis – lithium treatment. Lithium treatment is probably under-used in Norway and when prescribed patients do not receive sufficiently good instruction in following it. Ottosson (1989) emphasises that only a few patients with the melancholic syndrome which has led to suicide have received treatment which is adequate in relation to drug therapy. More effective treatment of major affective disorders could probably reduce the suicide rate in Norwegian institutions. There has certainly been too great a tendency in Norway to assess the disorders of patients from a psychodynamic point of view, and the more manic-depressive conditions have not been looked at sufficiently as disorders which are probably also biologically based and are often best treated with drugs.

No special programmes have been devised in Norway for the treatment of those at risk of suicide in psychiatric hospitals. Guidelines of this kind have been issued in Sweden by the National Board of Health and Welfare's Care Programme Committee (1983): 'The problem of suicide. Care programme documentation. Compiled by a working group directed by Jan Beskow'. This book gives more detailed guidelines both for treatment in psychiatric hospitals and clinic wards and in the primary health service but unfortunately only in Swedish.

Preparation for discharge – flexible institution arrangements

Discharge can never be planned too carefully. It should be done in co-operation with the family. It may occasionally be an advantage for the institution to be able to offer flexible transitional arrangements, in the form of day or night hospital stays.

In the *day hospital* the patient may be treated in the institution during the day but spend the night at home. Conflicts which arise in the home environment can always be dealt with as and when they emerge.

A *night hospital*, where the patient is at work during the day but spends the evening and night in the institution is often very suitable during a transitional period after discharge from the full-time ward. A night hospital may be suitable for lonely people who live in bedsits, who can cope with their jobs but cannot cope with the frustrating existence in a lonely bedsit through the evening and night. In the night hospital they are in the company of others whom they know to some extent from their hospital stay, during the evening and night.

The most important aspect, however, is the *after-care plan*. It is when the patient has to return to the day-to-day environment that provoked the suicide attempt that the need for outside help is greatest. It is probably also at this stage that the treatment apparatus is most neglected. All experience shows that it is in the first six months after discharge that the danger of suicide and a fresh suicide attempt is greatest. In the treatment of the suicidal patient in the institution there will always be a difficult balance between checking and supervision on the one hand and trust and freedom on the other. This will also be the case in the after-care situation. The patient attends for regular checks during after-care. The problems are discussed with him as they emerge. Simply for the patient to know that he has someone else to discuss his problems with may be enough to prevent a fresh attempt or suicide. The patient's dosage of medicine can be adjusted. Care is taken to ensure that he does not receive so much at once that he can commit suicide. It is particularly important to be aware of this problem when prescribing antidepressant drugs, where the difference between the fatal dose and the therapeutical dose is small. Co-operation must be established with the immediate family. The after-care plan may last for several years. It is also important for there to be one person with whom the patient is in contact over the course of time. It is unfortunate if the patient returns to find constantly changing therapists who did not know him or her previously, and with whom a relationship has to be built up on each individual occasion. There is an increasing awareness of the importance of continuity in treatment.

The restructuring situation that has arisen in many institutions in Norway has without doubt been unfortunate, although the intentions have been good and the restructuring will be beneficial in the long-term. Many patients have come to unfamiliar institutions when they have suffered a relapse, with a lack of the continuity which is vital to suicide-prevention work. It cannot be emphasised too strongly how important it is for patients to have familiar central persons they can relate to, and for them to enter a system where they feel welcome and which they can count on as being *theirs*. The constant changing of admission areas for the psychiatric clinic wards and hospitals which has been seen in Oslo among other places may have an unfortunate effect on patients at risk of suicide, who can easily feel rejected and less welcome, with tragic consequences. The trend seen in psychiatry in recent years for rapid discharge, particularly because of lack of space, has also been unfortunate.

It appears to me that the closure of psychiatric hospitals has proceeded too quickly, and that the shortage of secure hospital beds has become acute. This has been particularly detrimental to the worst psychotic patients and also those threatened by suicide. Alternative schemes in the community have not been built up to a sufficient extent. When psychiatric hospitals started to be closed down in the USA, the intention was that some of the clients would be caught by the mental health centers, many of which were set up. However, it was found that the mental health centers were less well equipped psychiatrically, and were directed more towards taking social clients and the easier part of psychiatry. The result was that the worst psychiatric patients, the chronic schizophrenics and others, remained outside, and instead had to spend much of their time homeless in the parks and subways of cities. Fortunately a situation of this kind has not been experienced in Norway. Great care should be taken to ensure that treatment is offered to the worst psychiatric patients, who often need more active treatment than nursing homes or out-patient clinics can give. The worst psychiatric patients, with chronic and persistent schizophrenic psychoses, make a substantial contribution to the suicide statistics.

Suicidal patients in a hospital ward

An account is given below of the guidelines drawn up in ward 6 B of Ullevål Hospital, in Oslo (from Jørstad, 1987):

(1) Psychotherapists and environmental therapists must always anticipate suicidal thoughts being present, and ask directly and openly about such thoughts. Explicit questions are also asked about what methods would be used, earlier attempts, in what situation the suicidal thoughts arise and whether the patient is afraid of losing control.

(2) When the presence of such thoughts is openly admitted, it is important that the patient is aware that suicide is regarded as an inappropriate act, since it finally destroys any interests and aims the patient has, and that the therapists want to do everything they can to prevent this.

(3) Suicidal thoughts can only be clarified and looked at as problems in an open and direct discussion. It is obviously important for both the psychotherapist and the patient to discuss the matter, and it cannot be accepted for suicidal thoughts to be something that is kept secret from the ward.

(4) The psychotherapists insist that both the patient and the therapist inform other people around them of the suicidal thoughts. This applies both to the staff and to the family. Suicidal thoughts must not become part of a therapeutic secret in a hospital, but must be talked about openly, and must be reported in joint meetings in the emergency ward (the admissions ward). Reports on new patients where suicidal thoughts are specifically referred to must be read every morning.

(5) A differentiated system is used for screening each suicidal patient, and for setting up a close relationship with a particular person. The ward is generally open, but can be closed if necessary.

(6) It is of the greatest importance in the ward to work systematically on counter-transfer reactions, particularly aggressive feelings which the suicidal patient often arouses among the staff. These feelings must be discussed openly in interdisciplinary meetings, in frequent specialist meetings and in meetings with doctors and nurses who take part in the guidance process.

(7) Post-mortem work. If a suicide has succeeded, it is important for the act to be discussed openly with the patients in the ward as soon as possible, and by the staff and at team meetings.

18

Should the treatment of those who attempt suicide be centralised?

There has been much discussion in Norway, as well as in other countries, as to whether those who attempt suicide should have their own special care, or whether they should be treated by the usual mental health service. In Norway the attitude has been that those who attempt suicide are to be regarded as psychiatric patients with a particular symptom, but usually also with other symptoms, and they are part of the group of psychiatric clientele which the health service should attend to, both the primary health service and the hospitals. These should, therefore, be equipped to cope with the special needs which the outward symptom of attempted suicide entails. In the sparsely populated country of Norway, this is probably a correct view. It will also be impossible to give specialists competence in suicidology if those who attempt suicide are not to be included in the routine treatment methods in general psychiatry and the general health service.

In some countries special units, for example suicide prevention centres, have been created for the preventive treatment of attempted suicide. It is in the USA in particular that such centres have been developed, spread across the whole country. The centres are manned by specialists – doctors, psychologists, social workers and nurses. A person can turn here if he feels in such a state that he may consider committing suicide, or if he has attempted suicide. He can first make contact by telephone, anonymously if he wishes, make an appointment or be admitted to an institution which co-operates with Suicide Prevention Centers. There is some favourable experience of these centres in the USA. In the Nordic countries there is only one such centre, in Helsinki. The most important function the suicide prevention centres have had is to increase competence in the subject of suicidology. Unique experience is acquired in such special units specifically with regard to people with suicidal problems. Much of the broadened knowledge we have acquired in suicidology has been obtained from Suicide Prevention Centers in the USA. They have without doubt played an important role on a world basis.

There are no separate suicide prevention centres in Norway because it is felt that patients with suicide problems should be treated within the primary health service or the mental health service, on an out-patient basis or as in-patients. However, it is debatable whether the time has now come for such a centre to be established in a densely populated region such as Oslo which could become a resource centre for the country for expertise on the problem of suicide. There is relatively little experience in Norway of this large and difficult specialist subject. One step along the way could be to set up a centre for suicidology, preferably with an academic link, so that suicide research could also have a base in a central institution in Norway. The development that has taken place in Norway, with a sharp rise in the suicide rate, might suggest that this specialist field should be strengthened by taking central measures. A national competence centre in suicidology is proposed in the national plan for suicide prevention (1992).

19

Special problems facing the bereaved after suicide

The situation may be more difficult for the bereaved after a suicide than for other mourners. This is due partly to the fact that suicide is not regarded as a socially acceptable way in which to die, and partly the tragic circumstances that have often preceded the suicide and have also affected the family. The aggression of which suicide may be an expression in individual cases against the bereaved and the feeling of guilt which many bereaved people will feel make the situation even more difficult. In the case of ordinary deaths it is easier for those around to commit themselves to giving consolation and looking after the family. After a suicide, close friends often withdraw, feeling anxiety and uncertainty, and often do not give the bereaved the support they ought to receive. For children bereaved by someone who has committed suicide the circumstances may be subject to taboo and be a subject which is not mentioned at any time in their lives. The bereaved will often harbour considerable aggression towards the person who has committed suicide, because he hurt them so much. They will also harbour a feeling of guilt, that they did not do enough, did not offer help, did not do what they could have to prevent the situation. There will always be plenty of opportunities to reproach oneself. However, this aggression will often be projected onto those around, so that the blame becomes attached to others. If the person concerned has been admitted to hospital, the aggression is directed not least against the attending staff. Doctors and staff are reproached, partly for giving the person in question too much freedom and partly for the treatment not having been good enough, and partly perhaps because the person concerned had been held in an institution. Just as deaths in most cases will induce a grief reaction which can develop into depression, so too and to a greater extent will suicide. The bereaved after a suicide are therefore in greater need of help in their grief than those bereaved after any other death. After a suicide has occurred in a hospital, attending staff should address the grief of the bereaved and also address the aggression which is naturally directed against the institution or the attending staff.

It may be assumed in most cases that the grieving is incomplete after a suicide. More support is demanded from those around in such cases, and specialists should be brought into the picture to a greater extent for those who have been bereaved by the suicide. After a suicide has occurred, the aim of the treatment apparatus in all cases should be to help the bereaved. The family will need support, the feeling of guilt needs to be addressed, and grieving must be carried out. In this way it will be easier for the family to be re-integrated into the world around and so be prevented from being isolated from society. A plan of treatment which is carried out success-fully in relation to grieving among the bereaved after a suicide will be capable of preventing psychiatric disorders later on, and also of prevent-ing suicide.

Suicide can be 'infectious'. There may be someone else in the family or in the vicinity who harbours such thoughts, where the suicide of one person can trigger suicide in another. The same phenomenon is also seen in hospitals. If there has been a suicide in a ward, a special watch out should be kept for signals from people who are in the danger zone.

20

What happens afterwards to people who have attempted suicide?

It is only in the last 20 to 30 years that we have obtained a proper answer to this question. The world literature has been full of scientific studies which shed light on other aspects of suicide and attempted suicide, and not least the background factors. The progression can only be clarified after a long time. It should be clarified by personal follow-up investigations, where those who have attempted suicide are visited and their subsequent fate is analysed, and their assessment of the attempted suicide after the event is also obtained. It is of interest to know whether the act has led to changes in the patient's life, in the social situation or in the person's relationship with the world around. However, this is a method of investigation which is costly in terms of both time and money. The mortality rate can be studied in a simpler way, through registers.

There is considerable experience of the personal follow-ups of psychiatric patients in Norway since it is a small country with a well recorded population. Many studies have shown how valuable such home visits can be. They allow us to see what the patient's environment is like, meet the patient's family, and usually achieve a better relationship with the patient. A follow-up of this kind should take place a certain number of years after discharge. The time perspective then comes into the picture. It is anticipated that at least five years should have elapsed since discharge before it is possible to make a reasonable statement on the progression of a psychiatric disorder. The longer the time perspective, the more correct the picture becomes. However, it is not favourable to wait too long, and after 30 to 40 years a large proportion of the patients will be dead. Such a long period of observation will also make it impossible for one and the same doctor to follow up the patient. A reasonable observation period will be five to ten years. It is an advantage if the same doctor is both the examiner and the follow-up examiner. The most favourable situation is for a follow-up investigation to be arranged while the patient is still in hospital. This type of investigation is known as a *prospective follow-up* investigation.

I shall consider later some of what is known about the subsequent fate of those who have attempted suicide. The information is taken from international literature. I have also worked scientifically on this problem, and in 1970 published a book simultaneously through Universitetsforlaget in Norway and Thomas in the USA on the long-term prognosis after attempted suicide. This book and my experience from this work form the basis for many of the assessments I make and also for the examples that are quoted. The study was based on patients admitted to the University Psychiatric Clinic in Oslo whom I had personally examined during their stay and for whom a follow-up investigation was arranged. This follow-up investigation was carried out after a period varying between five and ten years. It was thus a prospective follow-up investigation by one and the same doctor. I later undertook an equivalent follow-up investigation together with the psychologist Britt Strype (Retterstøl & Strype, 1973) of patients who had been admitted to Sandviken Hospital in Bergen and had attempted suicide.

Later suicide

In most follow-up investigation studies, mortality rates from suicide varying between 1.5 and 15% over the course of a period of between 2 and 15 years are found. The Swiss psychiatrist Schneider (1954) studied a group of hospitalised patients in Lausanne who had attempted suicide. He found that around 10% had died as a result of suicide after 10 years had elapsed. After 18 years the percentage had increased to 11.8, and after a further 10 years the percentage had risen to 13. This suggests that the risk of suicide is greatest during the first few years, and declines somewhat as the years go by. The Swedish psychiatrist Dahlgren did pioneering work as long ago as 1945 in the follow-up investigation of people who had attempted suicide (Dahlgren, 1945). In his study from Scania he found that 6% of the patients had committed suicide, all during the course of the four years after admission. He has been monitoring this group of patients for 35 years. In his paper published in 1977 on this same group of patients, he showed that the percentage who had committed suicide had risen to 11%.

The percentage who have died will obviously depend considerably on where the study group is taken from. In the group of patients from a psychiatric clinic, which chiefly has acute cases and not mental illness cases, the percentage will usually be lower than in groups from psychiatric hospitals, which usually have more severe and more long-term cases with serious mental disorders. In the two studies I have carried out, the suicide rate in the first study, which was from a clinic, was 2%, whilst the rate was 6% in the group from the psychiatric hospital.

There are now several follow-up investigations around the world in which the percentage of those who have died as a result of suicide varies widely from over 15% down to almost zero. The observation period varies greatly, however, from less than one year up to the long obser-vation periods of 28 and 35 years adopted by Schneider and Dahlgren.

In Norway in recent years (Rygnestad, 1988; Ekeberg, Ellingsen & Jacobsen, 1991) suicide rates of 8% in Trondheim and 13% in Oslo have been found – both after a five-year period, and both in poisoning case material from departments of internal medicine.

If a single average figure has to be given it can be anticipated that approximately 10% of those who have been admitted to psychiatric wards after suicide attempts will die through suicide later on. Expressed differently, 90% of those who attempt suicide do not die directly from the attempt, but eventually die from other causes. This is worth noting.

Let us look at an example of a patient who later died as a result of suicide.

EXAMPLE 1

At the time of admission, this male patient was 65-years-old. He had been the middle child in a family of seven in a strict and orderly childhood environment. After school he went to sea and spent a number of years on long voyages and coastal voyages until he married at the age of 38. He then returned to the shore and took over his father's business, which he then ran alone. The father died when the patient was 50-years-old. The marital relationship was described as good. He had always been obstinate and stern by nature, but was also gentle and generous. During the war he had been a passive member of the Nazi Party, and was heavily fined and served a prison sentence lasting a few years. His small business was closed during this time. He had been isolated from friends and family during the war, and was also isolated from them afterwards because of his term of imprisonment. He was bitter about the fate that had befallen him and tried to justify his conduct during the war in many ways. After he had served his sentence he took over the business again, but allowed his son to manage it and increasingly withdrew. He felt superfluous, became restless, did not feel at ease either at home or in the business. Five years prior to his admission he gradually became more dejected and was admitted to a psychiatric clinic where he received six courses of ECT for his depression. He recovered and started to work again. Two months before the new hospital admission, he went through a period of increasing dejection. On one occasion he waded out into a small lake to drown himself, but the courage failed him at the last moment, and he returned to the cabin he had come from. However, he said that he would like to try to put an end to it all. The depression increased, and he had to be re-admitted to the clinic. He received some further ECT, this time with no significant effect. On the wishes of the family he was discharged again after a few weeks. Shortly after being discharged he made a fresh attempt at suicide. He was re-admitted unconscious after having poisoned himself with tablets. He was transferred from the somatic ward to the psychiatric clinic. Here he was deeply depressed again and talked about his bitterness and the unjust treatment he had received. Moderate atrophy of the brain was detected. He recovered well under treatment with antidepressants, and was practically in a neutral state of mind when he was discharged to a rest home after a few months. Nothing was heard of him until it was reported six months after he had been discharged that he had committed suicide by drowning. The family was apparently not aware that he had begun to be depressed again, and the suicide came as a great surprise to the family. In this case it was a fairly severe depressive disorder which was manifested in several attacks which certainly had some connection with his isolation, war experiences and in his opinion unfair treatment by the courts. His age was also of decisive importance in that he had gradually moved outside the firm and his brain had also started to atrophy. He probably felt himself that he had got into a situation of which he could no longer find a satisfactory way out. This suicide could possibly have been prevented by better after-care provision, and by helping him to a more meaningful situation in the business, for example a peripheral but nevertheless meaningful part-time job.

Death from other causes

The mortality rate is generally higher in patients who have attempted suicide than in an equivalent group of the normal population. The increased suicide rate only contributes partly to this. Those who attempt suicide also have a higher mortality rate than others because of physical disorders, for example because some patients have simply carried out the act to escape from a fatal, chronic or painful physical illness. In addition, attempted suicide, as mentioned earlier, is often carried out by patients who abuse alcohol or drugs. These patients generally have a very high mortality rate. It must also be anticipated that suicidal patients may be more prone to accidents than others, because attempted suicide in some is a 'chance' they have taken, an expression of a tendency in their personality to take chances and let Fate prevail. Many of them exhibit what is known as risk-taking behaviour. In Norwegian case material Bratfos (1971) found that the mortality rate was eight times higher among those who had attempted suicide than among control patients. In case material consisting of psychiatric patients, Noreik (1971) found that out of those who had made suicide attempts prior to admission, some 10% were dead after five years compared with some 6% of those had not made such an attempt.

More recent studies confirm these findings, and show that the mortality rate is very high in self-poisoning case material, particularly if the abuse of drugs is involved. Ekeberg *et al.* (1991) found in a group of continuously admitted patients at Ullevål Hospital in Oslo that 122 out of 934 had died after five years, with a strong preponderance of deaths among abusers. Suicide accounted for 28% of the deaths, the remainder being divided between the following causes of death: opiate abuse (16%), heart diseases (14%), accidents (11%), alcoholism (9%) and others (22%). The standard mortality rate was greatly increased in all groups (eight times on average), and was highest among female opiate abusers – 63 times higher than expected. The suicide risk was 87 times higher than expected among women and 27 times higher among men. The factors which were most strongly correlated with death during the observation period were gender (men), age over 50 and lowest socio-economic group. Age over 50 and previous suicide attempts were most strongly correlated with suicide during the observation period. Rygnestad (1990) found a mortality rate of 13% after five years, 8% for suicide (number of patients 253). He found that the mortality rate was 109 times higher than expected among women and 73 times higher than expected among men – a significantly higher mortality rate than in the case material of Ekeberg *et al.* (1991) The increased death rates are certainly also an expression of the burden of mental disorders in these groups. Equivalent findings have been made in Great Britain (Hawton & Fagg, 1988).

Later suicide attempts

A certain percentage of the patients make 'unsuccessful' attempts at suicide again. These percentages usually vary from 40% down to 10%. An average figure will be approximately 20%.

The percentages quoted will probably generally be minimum figures. Mild attempts which have not led to admission may be concealed by the patient or the patient's family, even in those cases where a personal follow-up investigation has been undertaken. All scientific studies agree that it is in the first six to twelve months that the suicide attempt is repeated, and most of the suicides take place during this period. This is natural. Firstly, it may be assumed that the problems which led to the attempt and which were the background to the admission will be most pressing and will be present most during the initial period. The feelings are again repressed, and the reaction can be seen in the time perspective. Secondly, it is likely that the new drugs, both antidepressants and antipsychotics, can cause rapid and artificial 'healing' of a serious mental disorder. It has not been phased out in a natural way and can re-emerge after discharge. It is therefore very important for patients who have attempted suicide to remain under after-care.

Do patients use the same suicide methods again?

Broadly speaking, they do. However, in my case material half of the patients used new methods or a combination of a new and an old method. This means that the doctors have to be cautious in prescribing drugs in large doses to patients who have previously attempted suicide, even if this attempt was made by a violent or other type of method.

Some patients will make many attempts

For these people, attempted suicide can become part of the pattern of their life, something they resort to when they encounter resistance. Such attempts can also be very serious. The fact that a patient makes constant attempts at suicide which he survives does not mean that he will continue to survive in future. However, it is possible to get away from such a pattern of life, as is shown in the next example.

Many hospital doctors in medicine, surgery and psychiatry gain the impression that once a person has made a suicide attempt, he will continue to make further attempts. This is due to the fact that those of us who work in institutions tend to see the recidivists, those who keep coming back, and not least those who are chronic. But we lose sight of the many who do not return. Only scientific studies of the type I have described can analyse this problem.

Conclusions

The following conclusions can be drawn:

(1) Approximately 10% of those who attempt suicide will die by suicide during the course of their life.

(2) Approximately 20% of those who attempt suicide will usually in the course of their life make further unsuccessful attempts. Expressed differently, approximately 70% of those who attempt suicide only make this one attempt.

EXAMPLE 2

This male patient was 30-years-old at the time of admission. He came from one of the western fjords of Norway. His father had been a farmer. The home was strongly religious. His mother had previously had a demanding office job, but after her marriage she became a farmer's wife, which she did not like. She missed her previous work, often said that she thought the children inhibited her and in many ways gave an impression of coldness. The patient was the youngest of four children. He was good at school. He passed his examinations well both at school and at commercial college. He then worked in an office and reached a senior position which involved a great deal of travel. He had had an unhappy love affair at the age of 16 or 17, and had later been engaged for a short time, but over the last 10 years had had a number of homosexual relationships. He was tormented by migraines, for which he had been treated. He was usually a bright and cheerful man with a good ability to get on with people, and had abundant energy. Immediately prior to the first admission to the clinic he took a large dose of sleeping pills because of an annoying headache. He was admitted to a somatic hospital and transferred to the psychiatric clinic. He was severely depressed, and it was feared that he would make another suicide attempt. It was found that he had taken too high a dose of sleeping pills, and he had been moved to a psychiatric hospital so that he would have more time for treatment. He was there for eight months. During his stay he made another attempt at suicide, and was only just saved. After being discharged from the psychiatric hospital, he moved into a bedsit. When he was due to start work again, he became very anxious. He started taking drugs again, increased the dose, poisoned himself again and was re-admitted. An attempt was made to treat him with psychotherapy and he was discharged again, whereupon he again started abusing drugs, taking quite high doses. He coped with his office work for the first few years, but made another suicide attempt with drugs of the same type. He was once again admitted to a medical ward and transferred to the psychiatric ward. In this ward he made several relatively serious attempts at suicide. He was nevertheless discharged after six months. After being discharged, he again made several serious attempts at suicide with sleeping pills. He was re-admitted to a general hospital and transferred from there to a psychiatric ward and a psychiatric hospital, where he was this time kept for eighteen months. He was in a secure ward for six months. He also made a suicide attempt there, by slashing his wrist.

After this attempt he recovered remarkably quickly. He found work. Good social arrangements were made by the hospital. He got a good job in a town which was not his home-town, but not in a city environment.

At the time of the follow-up investigation, five years after he had been discharged from the last hospital, he was very cheerful. He had been in work without being off sick throughout this five-year period, was coping well with the job and was extremely content. He was still unmarried and living in a bedsit. He said that he thought life was worth living again. No-one paid tax more gladly than him, he said, because this was a sign that he was a useful member of society again. He did not abuse drugs, and his employer was very satisfied with him as a particularly dutiful and energetic man. He had not made any suicide attempts in the last five years. There was reasonable hope, therefore, that he would cope with the rest of his life without attempting suicide and without abusing drugs, if no unexpected circumstances should arise which would once again take away his enjoyment of life.

What happens to the psychiatric disorder?

It is not possible to make a general pronouncement on this. Attempted suicide is usually just one of many symptoms of a psychiatric disease, and the progression of this condition will obviously depend on the underlying disease. If it is regarded as schizophrenia, which may have developed insidiously and apparently without triggering factors, the prospects will be worse than if it is a depressive condition of a manic-melancholic or reactive type. Fortunately the attempted suicide is often an expression of a depressive condition. Experience shows that these progress favourably and are generally cured, although relapses may occur.

With regard to my own case material, I found that over half the patients from the clinic had coped without being re-admitted to a psychiatric institution. The others had been re-admitted, generally for a short time, and only 6% were in a psychiatric institution at the time of the follow-up investigation. The others were at home. These findings are in close agreement with those obtained by Dahlgren (1977) and Schneider (1954).

However, the case material from Sandviken Hospital (Retterstøl & Styrpe, 1973) showed that a third of the patients there still had significant psychiatric problems, although the remainder were regarded as having been cured or having improved. Sixty per cent of the patients from the psychiatric hospital, who were a more difficult group of clients, had been re-admitted to a psychiatric hospital or clinic during the course of the observation period.

An example is quoted below of a psychiatric disorder which proved to be chronic. This patient was in a psychiatric institution at the time of the follow-up investigation.

EXAMPLE 3

At the time of admission, this man was 45-years-old. He was the youngest of three children. The family had moved when he was six years old to the parish where he was living at the time he was admitted. There were many arguments between the parents, the mother occasionally left home to return to her own childhood home, and usually took the children with her. However, she always returned to her husband. At school our patient was an able pupil, and he later worked in agriculture and fishing. He was married 20 years prior to his admission to a woman from the parish in which he had grown up. He afterwards ran a farm owned by his wife. There were seven children from the marriage, who were aged between six and 19 at the time of his admission. The oldest two had left home. His wife was wealthy, since she had inherited a large amount of money. On the insistence of her father, the couple had separate property. The patient was almost to be regarded as a farmworker on the farm owned by his wife, where the patient's mother-in-law also lived. He felt rather 'left out' of the family situation, and was jealous of his wife, who was the strong partner in the marriage. The relationship between the couple was poor. The patient himself was a somewhat capricious man with fluctuating moods, sometimes quick-tempered and uncontrollable, at other times suspicious and jealous. He was a heavy drinker, without there being major alcohol abuse. His wife was very critical of him for this. A few years before the admission in question he had been admitted to a psychiatric hospital. He was finding it difficult to sleep, was restless, heard voices and thought his food was being poisoned. It was a brief attack. The wife had asked the local policeman to help her get the patient admitted. The patient had then threatened them with his gun.

Some time before the admission in question he again suffered the same symptoms. During a period of sleeplessness he disappeared, but after 12 hours was found in an out-building. He had cut himself quite seriously in the neck and had to be admitted to hospital. This time he was not transferred to a psychiatric clinic ward after the attempted suicide, but was sent home after his physical condition had improved sufficiently. Three weeks later he drank a whole bottle of chloroform oil, apparently in order to put an end to it all. He also expressed violent jealousy.

During his stay in the psychiatric ward it emerged that the marital conflict was serious, and that his wife had several times asked for a divorce, and that she had sometimes called the local policeman and doctor when the patient became difficult at home. It was clearly understood that he was not welcome at the farm and in the home. During his stay he appeared unresponsive and suspicious and trivialised his problems. No definite signs of mental illness were found. The impression was gained that the marriage would not work in the long term. He was nevertheless discharged and sent home. At home he made two further attempts at suicide in the following two years, one by slashing his wrist and one by taking tablets. He recovered both times, and was not admitted to psychiatric wards. However, considerable difficulties arose at home, particularly in his relationship with his wife and mother-in-law. After a few years he developed increasing delusions about being persecuted. He was admitted to a psychiatric hospital. The first time he was only there for three months, but each time he went home, his wife stated that he was impossible to have at home. He was admitted a total of five times to psychiatric hospitals in a fairly depressive state and with delusions. He has been in a psychiatric hospital for the last few years, and it appears as though he will have to stay there for a long time. He now has a well developed paranoid mental disorder.

What is social function like?

Most studies show that those who have previously attempted suicide later function well socially. According to my first study, 80% of patients were fully functional in society at the time of the follow-up investigation, 11% were in receipt of disability pensions and the remainder were receiving some other form of assistance. Dahlgren (1977) found in his case material that two-thirds of his patients were fully functional in society. A high figure for those who were fully functional in society was also found in Danish case material from Odense. However, only one-third of the case material from Sandviken Hospital in Bergen (Retterstøl & Styrpe, 1973) were fully functional in society. This again reflects the fact that this was a group more affected by problems, half of whom were diagnosed as having a psychotic illness.

What happens to young people who have attempted suicide?

Attempted suicide among young people is an increasing problem, as we saw earlier. The prognosis for these young people has been elucidated for example by the Swedish psychiatrist Ulf Otto (1971). He examined the entire case material from Sweden of people who had made suicide attempts and who were younger than 21-years-old – a total of 1547 children and young people. There was a preponderance of girls. He compared what had happened from a number of registers and assessed the case material against a control group. His observation period was 10 to 15 years. He found a strong preponderance of deaths among those who had attempted suicide and, as expected, a strong preponderance of suicides. He also found that the group of young people who had attempted suicide had in many ways developed differently than the control group. For example, fewer had married and those who had married had had their marriages terminated by divorce more commonly than the controls. They had emigrated from Sweden to a greater extent. They were in receipt of a disability pension to a far greater extent, had committed more criminal acts, had greater alcohol problems, and were referred to corrective schools to a far greater extent than the controls. Periods of sick leave were also considerably longer, for both psychiatric and physical disorders. They had performed their military service to a lesser extent than others. Those who had completed it had a less favourable record. In most respects they constituted a group which turned out worse on most variables than the normal control group.

View of the attempted suicide

Most patients who have attempted suicide are later pleased that the attempt did not succeed. In my study 75% were pleased that the suicide attempt at the time had not been successful. Other researchers have found similar figures. In my case material from Sandviken Hospital the percentage was lower – 57%. We can nevertheless safely state that most of those who attempt suicide are pleased that they have survived.

Of the patients with whom I was in contact at the time of the follow-up investigation of the clinic case material 17% told me that they had thought about making another attempt at suicide from time to time. This is certainly a minimum figure. However, most of them positively stated that they had not been occupied by such thoughts.

It is striking, however, that patients who have attempted suicide are not keen to talk about it afterwards. It is known that psychiatric patients are rarely keen to talk about their periods of illness. This is quite understandable, because they are usually associated with painful memories. The same is true of all of us. We would prefer to talk about the happy and pleasant memories from our lives, and try to push away the nasty and sad memories. It is perfectly understandable for a patient who has attempted suicide not to be keen to talk about it. To many people it is a miserable and shameful act, a sign of having failed to cope with day-to-day living. There are also many taboos. The act has also been related to a situation of difficult conflicts which the person in question has not been able to solve.

Factors of significance to the prognosis

I have already discussed the factors which suggest that the suicide attempt will be repeated and possibly that the patient will finally die by suicide. It is difficult to assess the danger of repetition in the individual case. As mentioned earlier, the mortality rate is higher among those who make a serious attempt at suicide, but the difference is not great. It can generally be said that the more serious the psychiatric disorder has been, the more this will be manifested in later mortality and also in the prognosis both clinically and socially.

Finally, mention must be made of factors of significance to the mortality rate, found in a major survey by two American researchers (Tuckman & Youngman, 1963, 1966), they found that the risk of suicide later was greatest among men, persons more than 45 years of age, those who are separated, divorced or widowed, the unemployed and old-age pensioners, the single, people with a persistent or chronic disorder, patients with nervous disorders, behavioural disturbances or alcohol abuse, people who had used 'tough suicide methods' and persons who had made serious attempts and left behind letters or messages. In their later study, which was considerably expanded in comparison with the first one, they graded the ranking order as follows: patients who lived alone, those who had used relatively violent suicide methods, those who had previous suicide attempts behind them, those who were more than 45 years of age, those who were men and those who had shown signs of nervous or mental disturbances.

There continues to be a lack of good follow-up investigation studies on those who have attempted suicide. These follow-up investigation studies should be made prospectively, that is the arrangements for the follow-up investigation should be made whilst the patient is still in contact with the hospital in connection with the attempt. A number of objective and subjective data which it is desirable to assess can then be obtained. This also applies, for example to the environmental therapy in hospital or what the therapeutic plan has been. All experience shows that it is very difficult to assess the importance of individual factors, and it is also difficult to assess the significance of a plan, even if it is structured. It will, nevertheless, be important to assess the significance of both the crisis intervention plan and the after-care plan. Follow-up investigations should be carried out in person, not by letter or over the telephone. If good evaluation work is to be organised, the consent of the patient to follow-up should be ensured. A follow-up investigation will be beneficial to the individual patient, and not least to our knowledge of the prognosis after a suicide attempt and what factors influence this prognosis.

21

What consequences does the suicide attempt have for the patient later?

This important question has received surprisingly little attention in the literature. There has been a clear awareness of the social effect of suicide attempts and suicidal threats. This has been expressed as follows:

> Suicidal threats permeate the whole of our social system. Suicidal threats force people to marry each other, prevent marriages being dissolved, force parents to turn a blind eye to the reprehensible behaviour of their children, delay admission to hospital, are rewarded by avoiding military service, have the effect that one child in a family may be favoured over another, etc.

It is only over the last 30 years that these factors in attempted suicide have been scientifically studied on the basis of personal follow-up investigations. I wish to illustrate this point with the experience I have gained in my own studies of patients repeatedly admitted to the University Psychiatric Clinic in Oslo.

It is common to all the patients that the suicide attempt was a major reason why they came under *psychiatric treatment* at the time. It led to the curing or improvement of the mental disorder in several cases. In almost one-third of the cases the suicide attempt was registered as *the most important factor leading to the patient's mental disorder being treated*. In a further third of the cases psychiatric treatment was instituted for the first time after the suicide attempt. It may be assumed in well over half the cases the patient was able to receive more appropriate treatment as a result of the suicide attempt. The suicide attempt functioned in these cases *as an alarm signal* which brought about hospital admission and treatment. It is likely that the psychiatric disorder in many cases would not have been treated if the person concerned had not tried to commit suicide. The disorder in some cases could have developed further and ended in suicide or a more chronic mental disorder.

For other patients, also around a third, the suicide attempt has been a decisive factor in their life. An event which had aroused themselves or their immediate family and changed something in their relationship with themselves and those around them. Some became divorced, possibly as a result of the psychological processing the attempt led to, in some cases the marital relationship improved considerably and for some important external measures were taken. This may be finding work, finding a home, and in some cases also the establishment of a long-term treatment situation. In around half the patients, the suicide attempt did not appear to have led to anything other than psychiatric treatment in an acute situation, no other significant changes having occurred. However, there appear to be important opportunities for help and improvement by being given treatment.

Let us first look at an example in which the suicide attempt was the trigger for a patient to come under psychiatric treatment for a quite serious case of psychotic disorder.

EXAMPLE 4

At the time of admission, this patient was 35-years-old, and worked as a domestic servant. There were several cases of mental disorder in the family. She came from a forestry environment and was the third of 10 children. The financial situation in the home had always been poor, and welfare bodies had had to help. She was kind and helpful and very sensitive when small. She coped well at school and later held a number of domestic positions. At the age of 17 she became engaged, but broke off the engagement herself. After which she had gone out with several men. Six months prior to admission it had been intended that she would get married, but there had been a hitch at the last moment, and the engagement was called off.

After this she found a job in a nursing home in another part of the country. She felt that the manager had it in for her. She became anxious and restless, wrote confused letters home, saying that she was being persecuted and was regarded as being a spy. It also appeared that she had auditory hallucinations. She was so tormented by being persecuted that she decided to go home. On the train home she became afraid that someone was after her. This caused her to suddenly jump out of the train window while the train was travelling at high speed, out of fear of her persecutors, on the grounds that it was better to die than be captured by them. She was admitted to a general hospital, where concussion and bone fractures in various parts of the body were found. After her surgical treatment had been completed, she was transferred to the psychiatric ward, where she was notable at first for her ideas of persecution. She was treated with neuroleptics, antipsychotic drugs. After a month she was discharged home. She has coped without a recurrence of her psychotic disorder, but she has had to stay in her home parish, still suffers from shyness and embarrassment and mixes little with other people. She has had occasional jobs in the parish. She talks a great deal about her suicide attempt and about the problems that preceded it. In this case it appears fairly certain that her suicide attempt was triggered by the mental disorder, and that it had been high time that she was treated for this. It is difficult to assess what would have happened to this patient if she had not come under psychiatric treatment at that time.

Let us now look at an example of a patient who also came under psychiatric treatment because of the suicide attempt, but in whom the treatment did not lead anywhere. The suicide attempt in this case led to a lengthy stay in hospital.

EXAMPLE 5

The patient was 40 years of age at the time of admission. There were a few cases of depression in the man's family. He was from a small holding with a poor financial situation and poor social conditions. The home was dominated by a silent, reserved father who had few friends, and who was very jealous of his wife. The mother was often ill with periods of depression and was admitted to a psychiatric institution several times. The patient was the third of six children. He was reasonably capable at school and helped at home on the small holding after he finished his schooling. He is depicted as a silent, bashful and unconfident man who easily gives up. Around 10 years prior to the admission, he went through a period in which he was at home for a year without work. He has been shy and bashful towards women. In the last year before his admission he had a relationship with a woman from a nearby town. This woman was divorced and had two children. She had become pregnant and told the patient so and suggested that they should get married. The patient was horrified about this and wanted to know whether she had been out with anyone else. He gradually became obsessed with this problem, and the potential paternity case. He became increasingly depressed and reproached himself for the wrong he had done. He had a feeling of perdition and disaster, and started to hear voices. One day he went into his woodshed and tried to hang himself. His father happened to be nearby, and heard something going on. He got the patient down from the rope just in time. The patient was so badly hurt that he was immediately admitted to a surgical ward, where he was just brought back to life. After his surgical treatment was completed, he was transferred in a very depressed condition to a psychiatric ward. He felt condemned and persecuted. He recovered well after being treated with six courses of electroconvulsive therapy and drugs, and was discharged home after the matter had been discussed with him and his family. He was re-admitted only six months after discharge. He had received a letter from the divorced woman and this had caused him to brood over the paternity again so much that he felt persecuted and believed that he was lost. He said that he could see no way out of the situation he had become entangled in. He felt on the one hand that it was his duty to marry the woman, but his parents strongly advised him against this, as did his friends, who disapproved of her and regarded her as an irresponsible woman. During his stay in hospital he was given a number of drugs, recovered somewhat and was tried out at home again. However, no solution to the problem with the woman was found and he was awarded paternity in a court of law. At home the symptoms worsened again and he had to be re-admitted to the psychiatric hospital where he has been virtually continuously for the last 10 years. He has become less interested in his acquaintances, and leads a rather passive existence. From time to time he is tormented by voices. He has not made another attempt at suicide. It appears that this patient is now suffering from a fairly stubborn and chronic mental disorder which is regarded as schizophrenia. Despite a long period of psychiatric treatment he has not been able to return to normal social life. It was the suicide attempt which at the time brought him under psychiatric treatment for the first time, but the treatment regimens in this case have unfortunately not led anywhere.

Around a third of the patients stated that the suicide attempt had been a *decisive factor* in their life, an event which had alerted them or their immediate family, and changed something about their relationship with themselves and those around them. It will always be difficult to say afterwards whether it is the actual suicide attempt or the underlying mental disorder which was decisive for the outcome. When there has been a favourable development, it will be difficult to decide whether this is due to the psychiatric treatment, including the psychotherapy, increased insight, whether there has been maturation of personality, spontaneously or as a result of the treatment, or whether chance external circumstances have played a decisive role.

Examples in which significant changes have occurred in the patient's life are given below.

EXAMPLE 6

At the time of admission this patient was 40-years old. She was a married woman from a labouring and fishing community. There had been a large family of 12 children. The home financial situation was poor. She was always sensitive when small. She attended ordinary primary school and domestic science school, and later worked in the fisheries firms in her home district. She then moved to an urban area in the same district and got married at the age of 25. There was one child from the marriage. There had been some problems in the marriage, particularly in her relationship with her father-in-law, who had lived at the property. She is depicted as a very sensitive and touchy woman, but with changeable moods, easily offended and angered. In the last few years prior to her admission her mood had been more unstable than it had used to be and there had been many aggressive outbursts. She had had the feeling that people were talking about her, and that rumours about her were being spread. She also thought that the whole of her husband's family where in league with him and were intent on making her mentally ill. When she was harbouring these thoughts prior to her admission she felt that everything had collapsed beneath her, and she made two attempts at suicide with tablets. Neither of them was so serious that she could not be treated at home. However, she was so down that she was admitted to a clinic after a few weeks. She had not previously been aware of her family problems. During her stay these were addressed. It emerged that there were considerable marital difficulties which had been going on for years. The recurring theme was the father-in-law, who was quite senile and whom the patient's husband had supported. Much of her conflict was at the family level. Her situation was addressed during her stay and her husband was brought into the picture. She went home again quite cheerful.

A follow-up investigation was conducted on two occasions, with an observation period of 10 years. After she went home, she took a part-time job outside the home. She talked to her husband about her father-in-law, and was allowed to break with both her father-in-law and her husband's family. The father-in-law later moved to an old people's home. Her husband at first thought this was a sad solution, but he realised that either the patient or his father had to move. The marital relationship became considerably better. She gradually started to mix with people in the district. Both the husband and her grown-up daughter expressed the view that the patient was much more cheerful than previously, and that a reasonable solution had been found to the family problems after treatment had been completed. They all together felt that the favourable development had been very closely related to the fact that the problem had been addressed after her suicide attempt. She had not had suicidal thoughts since, and was fully functional at the time of the follow-up investigation. The addressing of her problems has probably enabled her to put into effect the measures which were essential for the later favourable progression.

In others there has been a significant *maturation of personality* in connection with the treatment. An example of this kind is quoted below.

EXAMPLE 7

The patient was a 19-year-old girl who was attending school when she was admitted. She had grown up in a very strict and emotionally cold environment, and there had been a great deal of physical punishment. She had ten brothers and sisters and was herself the middle child. Her father was dominant and decided everything at home, whilst her mother was subjugated. When the patient was aged about 10, a sudden breach occurred between her parents when it was discovered that her father was having an affair with another woman. Her mother demanded a divorce and moved away with all the children. She initially went home to her parents. She then moved around the country in connection with various jobs she took. This led to the home being characterized by rushing, restlessness and a poor financial situation. The mother had little time to look after the children. The patient had always been clever at school. She had been sent by the mother to a junior secondary school noted for its very strict religious attitude. Although she was used to this strong religion from her mother, she now found it difficult at school. She felt that pressure was being put on her Christianity, and she did not always manage to live up to the expectations of those around her. She acquired a boy-friend – a fantasy boy-friend – during her time at school, whom she only saw to say hello to, but who she thought was deeply in love with her. Later she was converted and confessed that she was a great sinner who had not been steadfast in her faith. She was the subject of much discussion and was called in for a talk with teachers on many occasions. She developed two 'fantasy lovers', one very sensual and physical, 'sinful', and one with a strong religious belief. When she heard that one of these 'fantasy lovers' had become engaged, she slashed her arm. She lost a large amount of blood, leading to a hospital admission. She was later transferred to a psychiatric institution. Here she received considerable psychotherapy persuading her into numerous conversations in which her childhood situation, her relationship with her parents, her puberty and her problems in relation to the opposite sex and religion were discussed. Her mother also came in for a number of discussions. The patient worked on herself and her problems well and clearly benefited.

She has now been followed up for eight years and is recovering well. She is now married and lives in another part of the country. Her marriage appears to be a happy one. Her husband also comes from a fairly pietistic background, but they have both consciously tried to get out of this, and believe that they have found an existence which gives them more than they had before. The patient later explained that when she tried to commit suicide she was making a strong protest against the environment she was in. She also faced significant problems in relation to puberty and her inadequate adjustment to the role of an adult. She was very grateful for the addressing of her problems that had taken place in the hospital, where she got to know herself better. She believes that, thanks to her stay, she managed to break out of the environment she lived in and establish an independent existence in marriage and life in general. She has not made any further attempts at suicide or received any further psychiatric treatment. It may be assumed that the maturation of personality which she underwent has been connected in some way with her psychotherapy.

It can be seen that considerable help was given to the patient and also to the patient's life as a whole after treatment in connection with the attempted suicide. For some, the treatment has also given them the courage to seek help again when their condition has become worse. But there are many examples in which the attempted suicide has led to relatively little change in the patient's situation – altogether in around half of the cases. I shall now present a case where the progression became favourable in the long-term, but where it was hardly the stay and the treatment which led to this improvement.

EXAMPLE 8

This male patient was 40-years-old at the time of admission. He was the oldest of seven children. One brother had committed suicide. The home was depicted as a peaceful and good working-class home. However, when he was small he had been a nail-biter and was often ill. He was good at school and afterwards worked on a farm until he moved to a town where he was employed by a large firm. When he was 22 he married a woman who was seven years older than himself. There were no children from the marriage. His wife had abused alcohol and drugs for many years. She was repeatedly admitted to psychiatric and medical wards, she was in psychiatric hospitals and health resorts, and she committed suicide by hanging two years before the patient was admitted. He himself is depicted as a quiet and bashful man, but had already started to drink before his marriage, after which, his alcohol consumption rose. After the tragic death of his wife, he started to drink seriously. He gradually came to be regarded as a chronic alcoholic. He just managed to keep it in check so that he was not fired from his job. However, he acted drunk at his place of work on several occasions, which led to his being moved from one department to another. He felt that he was inadequate and started harbouring ideas that someone had it in for him, and that people were prowling around his house. He became more and more sleepless and nervous. Finally one cold winter's day he took a large dose of sleeping pills and jumped out of a first-floor window in the house. When he was found by some neighbours in the morning, they at first thought that he was dead. However, he revived after he was admitted to hospital. After he had been treated for two weeks, he was transferred to a psychiatric ward. His alcohol abuse and problems in life were discussed with him. However, he did not have the motivation to address his problems in detail. He himself believed that he would be able to sort out his affairs. Nothing in particular was achieved during the 14-day period he spent in hospital before he asked to be discharged.

A follow-up investigation was conducted eight years later. As might be expected, he had continued to drink heavily after his discharge. It so happened, however, that the following year he had started going out with a strongly religious woman from another part of the country, a lady who was both strict and well-intentioned and who clearly saw it as her task and duty to help him. She gradually become more central to his existence. Two years after his stay in hospital they married. He had to promise beforehand that he would not take any poisons in the form of alcohol and drugs. He coped with this. At the time of the follow-up investigation he felt satisfied with a successful marriage. He was working in the same job as previously. He was without doubt a 'henpecked husband', on whom his wife had quite a firm grip, but he had accepted his position. As far as could be gathered, there had not been a single recurrence of his alcohol problem during the time he had been married. The significant improvement which had occurred in this case is unlikely to bear any relationship to the suicide attempt, nor to the subsequent treatment. The result seems to relate to the later marriage, and the situation that he has subjugated himself to the authority of his wife.

It is apparent from the hospital case-histories quoted that the suicide attempt in some has actually been the only *alarm signal* which has given the push for medical and social treatment. Both the patient and the patient's family often find it difficult to seek help for the mental problems and psychiatric symptoms. It is easier to help when the patient has harmed himself, as after an attempted suicide.

An important factor after a suicide attempt may also be the *changed* attitude of the immediate family. Deep down, many members of the family are aware that the psychiatric symptoms may have something to do with themselves, for example the husband or wife in a marriage. They want to shelve the problems for as long as possible and not talk about them and hope that the whole thing will pass over. The suicide attempt can then come as the dramatic introduction to a 'purification process' which was necessary but which would not otherwise have been carried out. The suicide attempt makes it clear to the patient and his family that it is necessary to take such a dramatic step as to admit the patient to a clinic or a hospital. This will in any case have the temporary effect of separating the person in question from his environment. This temporary separation can enable the patient to put his life in greater perspective and also obtain help from specialists.

It is an important finding that a third of the patients have assessed the suicide attempt and the circumstances surrounding it as being a decisive factor in their life. Other colleagues have had similar experiences.

The fate-determining character of the suicide attempt

It appears that for many the suicidal act has been a kind of gamble with Fate. The situation has been hopeless, no way has been found out of it, and Fate has been gambled with. This aspect of attempted suicide is referred to as *the gambling character of the suicidal attempt*. The expression *the ordeal character* of attempted suicide has also been used. The term *Gottesgerichtsfunktion* (divine judgment function) is used in German – God is challenged. This could be translated as 'the fate-determining character of attempted suicide'. What is meant by this is that many patients feel that they have challenged Fate (God) in the suicide attempt, and in response have been allowed to hold onto life. They then accept this. As will be apparent from many of the case-histories, many patients have challenged fate in a very dramatic way. Only chance circumstances have saved them. It is striking how many of the patients who have made serious attempts have not repeated the attempt. The explanation may well be that they felt that they have challenged fate and have received their reply. However, it may also be that the depressive disorder which lay behind the act has been correctly treated. The most important basis for the suicide attempt has been taken away.

Are suicide and attempted suicide entirely different conditions?

It has previously been a fairly commonly held view that attempted suicide is either a failed suicide or just a hysterical demonstration. Many people believe that there are two separate groups of those who commit suicide and those who attempt suicide, but that there is some overlap between them. Evidence in favour of this comes from the earlier follow-up investigation studies which show that only a small proportion of those who attempt suicide later go on to commit suicide. However, many of those who commit suicide have previously made suicide attempts, and there is without doubt some overlapping.

The well-known British suicidologist Stengel has written that 'there is a social element in the pattern of every suicide attempt. If we look for this element, we can find it almost without any difficulty in most cases' (Stengel, 1967). He points out that those who attempt suicide have a *Janus face*, partly directed towards the renewal of human relationships and partly directed towards death. When the patient's life has been saved, it is the first aspect of the Janus face to which the eyes of the therapist must be directed. He must build on the will to carry on living which we have so clearly seen is present in our suicide attempters. Philosophers and poets have also been aware of this will to live in the person who attempts suicide. Schopenhauer expressed it as follows: '*Der Selbstmörder will das Leben, er ist bloss mit den Bedingungen unzufrieden, unter denen es ihm geworden ist.*' (The person committing suicide wants to live, he is merely dissatisfied with the conditions of his life.) The French poet, philosopher and politician André Malraux expressed his perspective on life as follows in *La Vie Royale*, '*On ne se tue jamais que pour exister.*' (One only kills oneself in order to live). I have seen this perspective on life take root so often in the patients I have examined and treated that I feel that it can serve as a motto for the whole problem of suicide. It also forms a natural point of departure for our treatment of the patient.

22

Deficiencies in the treatment of patients who are under threat of committing suicide

Unfortunately there are many major deficiencies in both organisation and the help mechanisms of today. Some of these deficiencies can be remedied by making an increased effort on the information front and through training programmes. It is often relatives, workmates, friends and other people close to the person concerned who can make the best effort when a situation in which there is a threat of suicide starts to develop. General education of the public on this topic is therefore important. Suicide has been an area very much subject to taboo, and if the taboos are to be broken down, it is important to discuss them. Many taboos without doubt still exist in the population. Many people look at those who commit suicide and those who attempt suicide as being of little worth, throwing away their lives or committing sinful acts. It has not penetrated deeply enough into the minds of the public that the problem of suicide is woven into human existence, and that each and every one of us may harbour suicidal thoughts, make attempts and even end our lives through suicide. The universal nature of the problem of suicide is something which people tend not to be aware of. There is, therefore, a need for public information and plenty of factual information campaigns on this topic, in the same way as public information is needed on the drug problem and psychiatry in general. It must be made clear to the population that people who try to take their own lives or harbour suicidal thoughts are people who have problems, crises, and who therefore have to be met with human contact. It is the near environment which is the best preventive factor. There is no doubt therefore that public information campaigns in this area are vitally important. We have far too few campaigns of this kind. The media have given insufficient attention to this topic, at any rate at the general level, and the specialists have not been clever enough or numerous enough to guide the population on this important area of human existence. However, it must be pointed out that sensational information can have the opposite effect, as we shall see later. The information must be sober and matter-of-fact the whole time, and not dramatise the situation.

If the public acquires this increased insight, far more help and warmth could without doubt be shown to the people in crisis with suicide problems. This in turn would lead to groups which are marginally concerned with the suicide problem also becoming better at providing help.

With the development that the problem of suicide has taken in Norway, in which ever younger groups are affected and there is now a large group of young people aged between 15 and 20, and since it is precisely in this part of the population that the increase has been sharpest, the time must have come for suicidology to be included in the teaching given in the school system. The problem of both alcohol and drugs has been introduced into the syllabus, and attempts have been made to give schoolchildren some understanding of the workings of the human mind. It may be sensible for schoolchildren at lower and upper secondary schools to be given instruction in this subject, as is now the case in the USA. This instruction must be given by the school's own people, the teachers, who know the pupils and can integrate the teaching of suicidology into areas such as the drugs problem, personality teaching and teaching on crisis problems in general. However, the teachers themselves have received little if any instruction in suicidology. This subject must therefore also be taught at teacher training colleges. If the understanding of suicidology is to reach out to the public, radio and TV programmes and press articles are not enough. The material must be learned from one's school-years, and those who are responsible for the teaching in schools must necessarily learn more about the problem than those who are to be taught.

Many occupational groups may need special courses. I am thinking here of ambulance staff, people in the rescue service, in the fire-brigade, police and prisons. People in the ambulance service, rescue service and fire-brigade are often in first-line contact with the suicidal patient, and many also need to learn how to tackle people with suicidal problems. Police officers are often present in situations where suicide is also threatened, perhaps in connection with alcohol abuse or what are known as domestic disputes, or disturbances or threats in public places. Police officers may often also be responsible for action which can represent a suicide-triggering factor, for example, arrest or confiscation of a driving-licence. Training programmes in suicidology must therefore form part of the training programmes for these occupational groups.

The social services are another social organisation which people at risk of suicide often come into contact with. They are the primary contact within society for many people. The social services often work with the groups at high risk of suicide, alcohol and drug abusers, people on the margin of society, and there is no doubt that the skills needed in dealing with people at risk of suicide could be increased within the occupational groups in the social services through education and training programmes.

Clergymen and congregation leaders are also people who are often confided in, including those who are threatening suicide. The problem of suicide should form an important element in studies and further training programmes for clergy and congregation leaders, and it is my impression that there is much room for improvement in the teaching on suicidology for these occupational groups.

We have previously discussed the central importance of *the primary health service*. There is no doubt that people who work in the primary health service as doctors, as doctors for parts of urban districts, municipal doctors, health visitors, nurses and social workers ought to attend training and refresher courses on tackling suicidal behaviour and the problem of suicide in general. My impression is that some improvement is taking place in this area. Courses in suicidology are held at various places in Norway, often run by the local medical associations, and lasting from half a day to one or two days, and interdisciplinary staff are also invited to attend these courses. Programmes of this kind are important in order that patients at risk of suicide are offered a better service and help. It must therefore be ensured that local bodies such as the local medical associations and also hospitals give training and refresher courses. It is important that these courses should not be one-off phenomena but are repeated at regular intervals. The staff changes, and new groups need information. It will probably be right to hold such courses annually.

The somatic hospitals, with their accident and emergency and intensive-care wards, also need regular instruction programmes. The service offered to those threatened by suicide may in some cases lag far behind what is desirable. A person with suicidal problems may have to sit waiting for a long time before psychiatric or human help arrives, either in a sterile room with a feeling of being in the way in a busy casualty department, where the person concerned may feel that he is a burden on the staff who are involved with other types of problems which are regarded as more important. In some places there is also a negative attitude towards patients who seek contact because of suicidal problems, perhaps associated with alcohol problems and perhaps also in an inebriated condition. People who at the outset were motivated to obtain help may lose courage when they have passed through so many hands such as ambulance drivers, an admissions office, a doctor for somatic treatment, nurses, and have gone from one door to another without their actual problems having been addressed. The energy required to live through this whole procedure can put a great strain on the patient's resources, and the patient may go away, slipping through the hands of those who give treatment.

If treatment routines are changed, a person could be made available who can remain with this patient throughout all these procedures. Some suicides might possibly then be preventable.

Somatic hospitals

We also looked earlier at the problems of the somatic departments when treating the actual suicide attempt. These departments are often intensive-care wards and service wards, where it is felt to be annoying and an imposition to have to give the person who has attempted suicide all the time and attention that may be necessary. Routines can be worked out in these wards where some continuity for the patient has been aimed for, and a particular member of the staff has been designated to have special responsibility for the person concerned, and if possible continuous 24-hour cover can be ensured by passing on information at the next change of shift. A great deal can be done in surgical and medical wards to improve the service provided for people threatened by suicide. It is valuable that several hospitals now have a consultant psychiatrist attached to them, who can give advice and help, assist in arranging the plan of treatment and not least arrange the course of instruction and strengthen the level of knowledge of suicidology in the department. It is important to work systematically on the matter through training programmes and try to find a better way of dealing with the many at risk of suicide. Research has shown that the staff in intensive-care wards have more negative feelings towards those at risk of suicide than the staff of psychiatric wards.

There are many major deficiencies in the mental health service. I shall now discuss these individual deficiencies.

The mental health service

Out-patient psychiatric treatment is not easy to obtain today. It is difficult for a person in need to get to see a psychiatrist or clinical psychologist. Most of those in private practice work to an appointments diary or offer psychotherapy by appointment, and are not available for people in acute need. It can easily become an ordeal for people seeking help with a suicidal problem. It is humiliating to turn from one doctor to another without being taken on by any of them. This situation can prove to be the last straw.

Psychiatric out-patients' clinics often also have a heavy work-load and are under time pressure, although they should represent the front line for this type of patient, and do so. It is important for it to be possible for appointments to be given at once, but it may also help for an appointment to be arranged for the next day or over the next few days. An example was given earlier in the book of a patient who without doubt made this serious attempt at suicide after receiving inadequate attention at the psychiatric out-patients' clinic, where no appointment was arranged, and which he had to simply leave.

The telephone may be useful in the out-patient situation. A request for a consultation may be the start of a telephone conversation which calms the patient down. Unfortunately the telephone is often regarded as causing a disturbance to clinical work. Many doctors, including psychiatrists, set aside telephone time which is very short, and it is often impossible to get hold of the key treating personnel when they are needed. However, the telephone is a good means of communication in such situations. It can be a great relief to patients to be able to confide in someone over the telephone or discuss their problems in this way. It is also a situation with less obligation for the person in question, who can even act anonymously and need not give his most intimate confidences. By giving over time to the telephone the therapist can do a very good job in the first instance for a patient threatening suicide. This resource has not been sufficiently developed in the treatment and prevention of suicide. The telephone also has the advantage that it can be used to discuss further plans, arrange a meeting or a home visit, and much valuable advice can be given. The psychiatric help system, both in out-patient units and in hospitals, should probably devote more attention to telephone work and use the telephone more consciously. People with suicide problems are a group of people who shy away from contacting others, but who can establish a relationship over the telephone which may be important in the situation and also later on.

The home visit is another form of treatment and examination which is used too little in psychiatry. Home visits can be of particularly great value in crisis situations. It can be easier for a patient who is in a state of panic and anxiety and has suicidal thoughts to be visited in his home than to take the initiative to travel to an out-patients' clinic or a hospital. Disasters can be prevented by a home visit of this kind. The home visit also gives better information on the individual patient and his immediate family, how he interacts with those around him and on his social situation. The real situation may be far more clearly apparent than in a consultation at the office or in an out-patients' clinic. A home visit is usually also appreciated by the patient as an expression of concern for and interest in him, and a more homely and personal relationship being created with the therapist or therapy team. The patient will also be more secure in his home environment and can present the situation more clearly.

Psychiatric hospitals and clinic wards also have deficiencies in their organisation of services for those threatened with suicide. It was pointed out earlier that the patient's mental and personal problems are often not analysed sufficiently in somatic hospitals, and that internal medicine specialists and surgeons also have to make an effort. An internal medicine specialist and surgeon can often meet a surly and unsympathetic response from the duty staff they contact in psychiatric wards if a transfer is considered necessary. Nor have psychiatrists committed themselves sufficiently to training programmes for doctors in somatic wards. Doctors out in the field as well as workers in somatic hospitals have found that it can be difficult to get patients into psychiatric wards or hospitals, and it can cost so much time and work that there may be a temptation to give it up. The psychiatric hospitals and clinics face problems of space. There is a particular shortage of secure places, as we saw earlier. The hospitals have presumably been too willing to reduce their list of clients, with the result that capacity has been over-stretched. Better coordination within the hospitals with the release of beds, particularly in secure wards, could lead to a more accommodating attitude on the part of the receiving psychiatric wards, which in the long-term could reduce the number of suicides. Fortunately, the introduction of the law on immediate aid has improved this situation. The psychiatric hospitals and clinic wards have a defined duty to receive patients who are considered to be in danger of taking their own lives. But small grants and resources, and perhaps also inadequate coordination, can make the situation difficult.

We looked earlier at the guidelines for the treatment of a patient at risk of suicide in the psychiatric ward or the psychiatric hospital. The guidelines are not always followed. There is a danger of important decisions today being taken with too low a level of competence. This is true of decisions on granting permission for patients at risk of suicide, for example to go out. There are clear guidelines for responsibility in a psychiatric hospital or a ward. It is the senior physician in the ward who has the ultimate medical responsibility, and he has to give his advice and instructions for the treatment, both in general and in the individual case. This responsibility may obviously be delegated. However, it must not be delegated too far down. *Major decisions in cases in which there is a threat of suicide should be taken by the senior doctor*, but outside of normal working hours is delegated to the duty doctor on call, who may need to seek help from the senior doctor. At most psychiatric hospitals arrangements have been introduced where doctors cover attendance duty around the clock, whilst senior doctors, in rotation, are available by telephone around the clock and can come in if necessary.

A great deal remains to be done within the psychiatric team to develop a sufficiently high level of competence. The assessment of people who have attempted suicide, or in whom the risk is considered to be great, should be made by a psychiatrist who has many years of psychiatric experience, including a good knowledge of suicidology and crisis theory. Psychologists, social workers and nurses can also become good helpers in this assessment through training programmes.

Regardless of how capable the senior physician and the psychiatric team are, it is not possible to avoid experiencing suicide in psychiatric wards and hospitals. This was explained earlier in the book. When a suicide occurs, it puts a great strain on all the staff who have been concerned with the patient, the ward as a whole and also on the other patients. It is important for a situation of this kind to be worked through thoroughly. It is in fact a form of grieving that is needed, both for the therapists and ward staff, and to some extent also for the patients. When such unfortunate events have occurred, meetings should be held among the treating staff to talk through the situation. What was done and what was not done? What could have been done to prevent this situation? It is also important for the patients to be involved in discussions, or at any rate to be given information. The family of the deceased must be brought into the picture and talk to the therapist and preferably the staff as well. There is a great feeling of guilt in situations like this, both among the therapists and assistants, and not least among the members of the family themselves. Family members tend to display aggression against the therapist, nursing staff and the hospital in general. This aggression should be addressed. A hospital chaplain can also be of great assistance following a suicide. A suicide can give rise to a crisis reaction in the family of the deceased, which in turn may also entail a risk to them. It is important to take time to talk to the members of the family. There are significant deficiencies in many hospitals in this area.

If a suicide has taken place in a ward or a registered patient has committed suicide whilst out on leave or while he was the hospital's responsibility, notification of the suicide and a description of the circumstances surrounding it have to be sent to the Directorate of Health, the hospital control committee must be informed and notice of the death must also be given to the police.

On the basis of the experience we now have, there is no doubt that work following suicides in the wards has often been given insufficient attention particularly in Norway.

Compensation matters can emerge afterwards. If the hospital has given reprehensible treatment, if guidelines have not been followed, or if serious errors have been made in assessments, compensation may come into question. There is an implied risk of suicide in psychiatric disorders, just as there is an implied risk of death in connection, for example with physical disorders or surgical interventions. Due care obviously has to be exercised by the hospital.

The staff at every hospital and every clinic ward must be given sufficient training and information on the problem of suicide. In most hospitals internal instruction and courses are given. It should be ensured that a course or a training programme in suicidology is given *at least* once per year, *or* as often as necessary, because new members of staff regularly arrive and have to share in the knowledge that exists in this important specialist field. It is also necessary for the older members of staff to have refresher courses provided and to have access to new material. Instruction of this kind should be given firstly at hospital level and secondly at ward level, and probably also at post level. The instruction should be given by teachers who are competent within the specialist field of suicidology.

Finally it must be mentioned that the assessment of the problem of suicide in the individual patient must also form an important part of the problem of teaching supervision. In hospitals the supervision of younger doctors in the training system with senior specialists is obligatory, and psychologists and nurses also have a supervision system which ought to make it possible to reduce the number of suicides. However, both the supervisors and those who are to be supervised need more instruction on the subject of suicidology.

Suicidology is a subject which is developing constantly. Every member of the psychiatric team must keep up with this specialist field. The International Association for Suicide Prevention and Crisis Intervention is an international organisation whose main topic of interest is the prevention of suicide. This will be discussed in more detail later in the book. It would be an advantage if more people in both Norwegian and European psychiatry and related disciplines were involved in this important international organisation.

23

Preventative measures

Earlier in the book I described a number of causes of suicide and attempted suicide. It could be said in a simple way that preventing suicide and attempted suicide involves removing the causes. This obviously cannot be done at a stroke. On the other hand, we cannot sit idly by and regard suicide and attempted suicide as an unavoidable phenomenon of society. The problem is very much like that of road accidents. In the mechanised and motorised society we live in, it is inevitable that road accidents happen. In many ways we can prevent them through social measures and educational activity. The roads can be improved, signposting improved, cars improved technically, technical checks and police checks can be made more frequent, laws on drinking and driving better enforced and above all there must be continuous education. This takes place for example through traffic items in the media, training programmes and tests. A great deal is done to reduce the number of road accidents. Nowadays twice as many people die by their own hands than in road accidents. However, little systematic work is done to prevent the major human and social problems which follow in the wake of suicides and attempted suicides – a great deal of work remains to be done here in society.

Primary prevention

Primary prevention means socially oriented measures which have a longer-term effect. All measures capable of contributing to a harmonious development of personality are subsumed under this heading.

These in particular include good, secure and harmonious relationships in the first few years of life, that is in the childhood home. If one of the parents is absent in earliest childhood without there being a secure substitute figure, the basis for an anxious and uncertain personality and for problems of identification is easily created. Growing up without parents, with only one of the parents, with constant strife between the parents, or constant moves and uprooting are circumstances which make it difficult for a harmonious personality to develop. The more warmth, love and security a child can receive in its first formative years of life, the better equipped it will be to cope in the difficult world people have created. Parents are generally not aware of the vital influence they have on the future mind and personality development of the child and of the possibility of making the child more or less predisposed to later mental disorder. If it is considered what an important and difficult role the parents have, it is striking how little society does to qualify its members to become good parents. Abuse of drugs and alcohol will always create problems in the nuclear family and in relation to the generation growing up. Fighting the drug and alcohol problem is part of primary preventive work, including the prevention of later suicide. An alcoholic home is rarely a happy home, and will always be an obstacle to developing people with a harmonious personality structure.

It can be difficult to identify how to make homes function normally. Many unwanted pregnancies and marriages could certainly have been prevented by *good* sex education and *guidance* on contraception. There is a long way to go until this education and guidance have been developed to a satisfactory level. Marriage guidance is uncommon in Norwegian society. Training is required for most professions but no training is required to enter one of the most demanding areas of society we have – marriage. Neither a knowledge of the laws applicable to marital relations, rules which ought to apply, or of problems which experience shows to arise is required. Nor is training required to enter the most responsible occupational role society has – the position of parent, a person who brings up children. *More* guidance on family formation and family life certainly ought to be included in school education.

Problem families and those known as *multi-problem families*, that is those who have many types of problems, constitute a disadvantaged group in society. They receive little help from society until very late or when it is already too late.

If problems arise in the marriage, there are few sources of help to turn to. There are some *family guidance offices*, but these are few in number and are not imprinted on the consciousness of the population. If the marriage has reached a stage where divorce is imminent, society provides a mediator, but his effort is of a formal nature. There is no team of specialists ready to help in situations which can be so decisive for the future of the couple and perhaps even more so for that of the children. Young parents do not receive, for example training in bringing up children or education in child psychology. However, in most places there are baby check-ups for very small children. This check-up has so far mostly been restricted to giving a physical service, measuring and weighing children, vaccination, advice on health matters and so on. There ought to be an opportunity at such check-ups to give guidance, including guidance on the emotional problems that follow from the role of a spouse and parent of small babies.

Society should also be able to make its services available later in childhood. The effort of the parents is particularly important in the first few formative years of life. Society ought to give mothers and fathers a better opportunity to be at home with the child in these important years.

Other social experiences can to some extent 'repair' some of the damage caused in the first few years of life, for example experiences in crèches and nurseries with new authority figures and other children to relate to. Children who come from a particularly difficult background need extra affection and care. The expansion of good nurseries with good specialist manning to deal with children from difficult backgrounds will also have a preventive effect on suicidal problems later, not least in adolescence.

A great deal can be achieved through *schooling*. An understanding and warm-hearted teacher can do much for a child if he knows how to assess the pupils individually and treat them accordingly. It is particularly important that no one should be portrayed as a loser or as inferior if they do not perform well at school. Everyone has areas in which they can assert themselves, whether it be gymnastics, mathematics, art or social studies. As mentioned earlier, in my opinion it will be natural to include knowledge of our personality development, and the many dangers we face of being derailed, for example through drug abuse, alcohol abuse or suicidalness. The problem of losers must be kept constantly in mind. They are to some extent the victims of our efficient welfare society. It is from their ranks that the young drug abusers and future alcohol abusers are recruited, as well as criminals, and those who later experience the problem of suicide.

Adolescence is a difficult time. Information campaigns and many provisions are still lacking. Recreation clubs, hobby clubs, sports clubs and associations of a religious, social, political or specialist nature can be of great preventive value. Adolescents need targets to work towards, commitment and the possibility of self-realisation. In adolescence too, those who have a good and trusting relationship with their parents and who have a homely base are best equipped. Young people who are poorly equipped in relation to their home life are unfortunately also the ones who have the least contact with voluntary organisations.

Special social groups require special effort. This applies in relation to the problem of suicide, particularly to such groups as those with alcohol and drug problems, people with deep depression, people who belong to minority groups and not least prisoners (see also section 'Secondary prevention').

Decentralisation measures come under the heading of primary prevention measures. Politicians in Norway have been very clever at aiming for a spread of the population and the maintenance of the hamlet-based social structure. There has been less of a tendency towards the break-up of local communities in Norway than in equivalent countries with which comparisons can be drawn, this is partly due to active decentralisation measures in political decisions. It is to be hoped that an effort can be made centrally for Norwegian society to be able to maintain its dispersed pattern of settlement and for jobs to be created locally according to a principle of decentralisation. District expansion measures can be regarded as a positive measure from the point of view of suicide prevention.

Measures with a view to improving conditions for the elderly and preventing them from being isolated are of great significance in suicide prevention. It should be borne in mind the significant development that has taken place for the very oldest age groups – those aged over 80 – where the increase in the suicide rate has actually been greater in the case of men than among young people.

In future we will without doubt have to give priority to measures to *increase* contentment among the elderly. It is also important for people to find a meaning in life outside of contentment and well-being, religious belief, political conviction, something to fight for, believe in and get involved in. Perhaps society has become too streamlined and an insufficient challenge for initiatives from individuals.

The level of unemployment in Norway today (1992) is unfortunate (the unemployment rate is now about 5%) and also predisposes to suicide, not least among the young. In addition to the registered unemployed anticipation has also to be given to hidden unemployment. We must not forget that it is youths from the least resourceful backgrounds who fail first in the fight for work and social benefits. Many young people who are unable to find work can be branded both in their own eyes and in the eyes of others as incapable, and lose self-respect and esteem. The percentage of losers easily mounts. Nationwide measures to prevent the consequences of economic downturns, unemployment and social misery will indirectly be important preventative measures with respect to the problem of suicide.

General educational work is one of the measures assumed to be capable of having a preventive effect in the long-term. Suicide in our society is a taboo subject. It is generally an advantage for taboos to be broken down and for it to be possible to talk openly about such subjects. This will make it easier to admit to suicidal thoughts and seek help, and also make the situation easier for those who are to help. It is important therefore for a subject like this to be capable of being treated in the media. On the other hand, publishing detailed descriptions and names in spectacular cases of suicide as occurs in some of the world's press must be avoided. Sensationalist coverage, on the radio and TV as well as in the press, seems more likely to predispose to suicide than prevent it. A separate section (p. 225) is devoted to suicide and the media.

Central health authorities can also contribute towards a reduction in some forms of suicide by introducing restrictions on access to drugs, which experience shows to be used in suicide. As mentioned earlier in this book, several important barbiturates were de-registered in 1980, with the result that a remarkable drop in cases of poisoning with barbiturates occurred. However, antidepressants have been seen to take over instead as the most important drugs involved in poisoning. Antidepressants are generally highly toxic, but developments are under way to put less toxic substances on the market. It appears that regulations from the health authorities have more of an effect on which drugs are used in suicide than on the actual rate of suicide itself. This approach to suicide-prevention should, nevertheless, *not* be abandoned.

Secondary prevention

These are measures which are directed against risk groups in the population who have shown a tendency to develop a disorder or who have perhaps already presented symptoms. In this case it is those groups of the population in which the risk is known to be particularly high. I have already discussed these groups and a number of measures elsewhere (see for example chapters 7, 10, 12).

Those closest to the person will very often be able to give valuable help *before* a suicide attempt is made. Education in general and guidance from specialists have great tasks to perform here. Friends and relations who can take time to talk to the person in question and lighten the burdens that seem to be unbearable are perhaps those who can make the best contribution to preventing suicide. General practitioners bear particularly great professional responsibility for helping people in crisis situations. It is, however, difficult for them to provide the optimum service to those who attempt suicide in terms either of training or time. It may be assumed that interdisciplinary health teams, in which psychologists, nurses and social workers work in close co-operation with doctors, can perform good work in suicide prevention. It is to be hoped that sectorised psychiatry can be developed further and become capable of intervening much earlier, including in the patient's home environment. It is also to be hoped that a greater degree of continuity can gradually be achieved in therapy and that people in crisis being shifted from one institution to another and exposed to the 'revolving-door policy' in hospitals will be avoided. Sectorised psychiatry and the primary health service are of central importance for establishing contact with people in the risk group.

As we saw earlier, people with depressive disorders, particularly of the melancholic form, are especially at risk, as are people with drug and alcohol problems and people in crisis in general. It is important to be able to establish diagnoses in the primary health service and intervene in relation to depressions earlier on and with a more correct method of treatment. *Increased knowledge of melancholia and its disguises and the melancholic equivalents* is necessary for all general physicians and non-psychiatric specialists, so that effective treatment can be instituted in time. It is also important for knowledge on the medication to reach all groups of doctors, since experience shows that there are groups of doctors who use too low a dosage of antidepressants.

Do we need separate institutions for the treatment of those threatened by suicide?

This problem has been discussed in chapters 17 and 18. Suicidal threats and acts are symptoms, and must be seen in relation to the other psychiatric symptoms and the life situation. The people concerned are in distress and have psychiatric problems. I believe that the better the psychiatric service apparatus that can be achieved, the better those threatened by suicide will be helped, and that suicide can be better prevented. This does not mean that it might not be appropriate to establish a central suicide prevention clinic in the form of a Suicide Prevention Centre, the principal tasks of which would have to be to raise the level of knowledge and research in suicidology.

Alternative provisions

The SOS service of the Church

A crisis intervention programme called *Telephonenseelsorge* was introduced in Germany in the 1950s. This church telephone service was jointly introduced by the Catholic and Protestant churches. In 1980 there were 68 such centres in Germany, taking around 200,000 calls. In the Nordic countries this service was introduced for the first time by the Swedish pastor Bernsprång, who placed an advertisement in the newspapers under the headline 'If you want to take your own life, phone Pastor Bernsprång.' A well developed network of SOS centres, which are open 24 hours a day, have gradually been created in Scandinavia. These SOS centres are spread around a number of large towns in Norway. The Home Mission has established an SOS centre in Oslo manned by more than a hundred volunteers day and night. The volunteers are people from various occupational groups who have followed a course. They are mature people who are willing to be on duty to help people in distress. People can turn to these centres when they are faced with a crisis, anonymously if they wish, and discuss their problems with people on the other side of the fence. It can help a person to find himself and can put him in touch with someone who can listen and give advice. It may be enough to make a person change his mind about his intention to take his own life. People of all religious views can turn to these centres, including those who have no religious interests at all. The Church SOS Service is not peculiar to Norway. There is an international organisation, IFOTES, which among other things holds regular international meetings and congresses, and which has also organised participation in the International Association for Suicide Prevention.

Other Norwegian provisions

The types of organisations presented here are found throughout the western world.

Alcoholics Anonymous (AA) is a grouping of women and men who try to solve a common problem by sharing experiences, strength and hope, and thus help each other to overcome their alcohol problem. The members work in groups which exist in most areas of the country, and have contact telephone numbers which can be used to obtain help.

Crisis centre/crisis telephone. There are crisis centres and/or crisis telephones in a number of municipalities. The crisis telephones offer conversation and advice and refer callers to a doctor, social services office and other public offices. They can also help to contact the police.

The Samaritans – the British approach

In Britain there is a suicide prevention organisation which does not exist in Norway – *The Samaritans*. The Samaritan movement was started in 1953 by Chad Varah, a vicar in a small parish in London. It is mainly based on telephone contact. In 1975 there were 165 centres in Britain, which took a million calls from 210,000 persons. The movement has grown over the intervening years, and has also spread to other countries. It is run in accordance with the 20 principles of the Samaritans. The key word is *befriending*. In this organisation there are volunteer helpers the clients can turn to. These volunteers have attended a course and are guided by specialists. There are more than 30,000 Samaritans spread across Britain, particularly in the large population centres.

An important aspect of the treatment is the friendly and compassionate attitude which the volunteers show in their entire behaviour towards those seeking help. The Samaritans offer friendship, neighbourliness and care. They are available by telephone at all times of the day. In cases where they think medical help is needed, they try to encourage the caller to visit a doctor. They have special medical contacts and guides, an organised supply of guidance both centrally and locally, with psychiatrists as guides. The well-known British suicide researcher Erwin Stengel was the central guide for the movement for many years. It is advertised with telephone numbers. The Samaritans put great emphasis on human integrity. Everything that is said is confidential. Each local department is led by one or more managers who are supported by medical advisers and consultants, so that the quality of the work can be as high as possible. There are systematic training programmes and those who are taken on are carefully screened beforehand.

The Samaritan movement has proved to be a healthy element in society in the direction of organising self-help. The organisation has been very positively received by specialists, both psychiatrists and other doctors. Attempts have been made to assess the effect of the Samaritan service. Suicide figures in towns where a Samaritan service has been set up have usually shown a downward trend. Many people see the fact that Great Britain is one of only two countries in Europe where the suicide rate has fallen in recent years as being explained by the extensive Samaritan movement and the work they perform there.

Suicide prevention centers – the American approach

The first suicide prevention programme in the USA was the National Save-A-Life League from 1906, started by Harry M. Warren under the auspices of the church. A telephone service was established in the form of a round-the-clock service for people in crisis, and still exists today. The centre is chiefly manned by laypeople with specialist guidance. It exists today in the Episcopal Church Center in Lower Manhattan (Hendin, 1982). There are now over a hundred suicide prevention telephone service programmes run by the church in the USA.

However, suicide prevention programmes were modest and attracted little public attention before 1960. In 1949 and the years that followed, Shneidman and Farberow performed fundamental research into suicide. This research work formed the basis for the Suicide Prevention Centers, of which a few hundred were eventually set up in the USA. The first was the Los Angeles Suicide Prevention Center, which was established in 1958, and the managers where the suicide researchers, Edwin S. Shneidman, Norman Farberow and Robert Litman, who were later to become so well-known. Shneidman and Farberow first received grants for their research from the National Institute for Mental Health (NIMH), and became increasingly concerned with therapeutic measures. The Los Angeles Suicide Prevention Centre was established with support from the NIMH, and was formed as 'an independent, nonprofit foundation and expanded into educational and training activities as well as clinical and research efforts'.

This centre formed the model for the more than 200 centres that gradually developed in the USA. Most programmes consist in making it possible to get in touch at any time of the day or night with a specialist who can make a referral for treatment for the person in crisis. This referral may be for a consultation or advice to a Community Mental Health Center, or for admission to a hospital or clinic. The programmes depend on a voluntary service where the telephones are manned most of the day round. Studies indicate that laypeople can function very effectively if they are adequately training and suitably guided.

Experience from Los Angeles has shown that virtually all telephone calls received are serious and come from people in distress. Around a third of the calls come from people who are not in immediate danger of suicide but are nevertheless in difficulty. Around 10% come from people in moderate to severe danger of suicide, and of these one in six are on the verge of death. The centre functions as a kind of mediation centre. Great emphasis is put on thorough training programmes for staff and on establishing a good environment. The large centres have professional administrators and paid therapists and laypeople for advice, and volunteers for part-time work and night-time work. These volunteers may be medical students, nurses, housewives, etc. Around a third of the centres are small and do not have any paid staff, a third only have one or two paid members of staff and the rest are voluntary. There is thus a significant difference in quality in the various centres. Doubts have been expressed over the effectiveness of some of the centres.

The suicide rate in 25 towns which did not have such programmes was compared with 17 towns which did have them. Over an eight-year period (1960–68) there were no significant differences in the changes in the two sets of towns (Directory of Suicide Prevention Facilities, 1969). David Lester (1974), who pointed out that the towns with centres were larger than the towns without centres, made a corresponding study by comparing towns of the same size. He did not find any significant changes in suicide rate in towns with or without Suicide Prevention Centers either.

Although research data does not appear to prove conclusively that the centres are effective in reducing the suicide rate, there is no doubt that the leading centres, primarily in Los Angeles, have had an enormous effect in furthering our knowledge of suicidology – fundamental scientific work has come out of these institutions, and all the people referred to above are in the top bracket of suicide researchers in the world. Suicide Prevention Centers modelled on those in America have now been formed in Germany, Switzerland and Finland (formed in 1972 in Helsinki). It is being considered whether a centre of this kind ought to be established in Norway to develop expertise in the area, for educational activity and not least to stimulate interest in suicide research.

Central European measures

Most suicide prevention measures have originated in Central Europe. In 1910 the urban mission in Berlin began its suicide pastoral care and a scientific conference was organised in Vienna, under the auspices of the psychoanalysis association of Vienna under the direction of Alfred Adler. Freud took part in the discussions. Suicide among students was the topic. The reason why the conference was held was the constantly rising suicide rate observed among students. School epidemics were described. However, no scientific work was presented at the conference, nor were any programmes put forward.

However, Vienna has been at the forefront with regard to suicide prevention work in the twentieth century. In 1927 an 'ethical community' (*Ethisches Gemeinde*) was set up in Vienna, aiming in particular to help people who had thoughts of suicide. In 1928 the philanthropist Wilhelm Börner, who was also the founder of the ethical community, set up a place for those who were 'tired of living' (*Lebensmüdestelle*), which gradually attracted around 60 volunteers. Among well-known names in this circle, Charlotte Bühler and Viktor Frankl can be mentioned. They set themselves the aim of working preventatively so that suicidal acts could be avoided, and aimed to co-operate with institutions that worked with young people. The work in Vienna aroused international interest. Similar measures were taken in Hungary, Germany and Czechoslovakia. These refuges for people in desperation were run until 1938, when the National Socialist movement opposed them and in some cases closed them down. During the Nazi period suicide was regarded as a natural 'purification process' in the people, by which 'inferior individuals' destroyed themselves.

Ten years after the war Erwin Ringel founded a suicide prevention centre in Vienna in co-operation with the Catholic Church and the Catholic welfare organisation Caritas. A team consisting of psychiatrists, social workers, doctors, psychotherapists, psychologists, lawyers and pastoral carers was built up. The suicide prevention centre was given the name *Lebensmüdenfürsorge*. Ringel was working at the time as an assistant physician at the University Psychiatry and Neurology Clinic in Vienna, and established a kind of personal union between 'Lebensmüdenfürsorge' and the university clinic. An agreement was reached under which all patients who had attempted suicide should be admitted to the detoxification ward of the University Psychiatry Clinic. After-care after discharge was usually given by Lebensmüdenfürsorge. This procedure was usually referred to in the literature as the *Wiener Weg der Selbstmordverhütung* (the Vienna way of suicide prevention). The falling suicide rate observed in Vienna was assumed to be due to the good service given to those at risk of suicide.

The work in Vienna without doubt formed the basis for the foundation of the International Association for Suicide Prevention, which has since had its general secretariat in Vienna. However, significant suicide prevention work has also been carried out at other places in Europe. Among the best-known is the centre in Berlin established by the doctor, theologist, psychologist and educationalist Klaus Thomas – *Lukas-Gemeinschaft, Lebensmüdenbetreuung*.

International Association for Suicide Prevention and Crisis Intervention

This international organisation in suicide prevention measures was founded in Vienna in 1960 on the initiative of the Austrian psychiatrist and suicide researcher Erwin Ringel. He arranged a European conference on suicide research in Vienna in that year. The proposal to establish an international organisation was at first met with some reservation when the association was founded on 17 September 1960. It is one of the few associations to have been formed first on an international basis, whilst national branches arose later. The opposite sequence is more usual. This organisation now has national associations in 35 countries. The largest of the national associations is the American Association of Suicidology. The organisation has held world congresses every other year since 1963 (when the international congress was held in Copenhagen). The congresses have tended to be held alternately in Europe and other parts of the world, chiefly America. The congresses have been held in Vienna (1960), Copenhagen (1963), Basle (1965), Los Angeles (1967), London (1969), Mexico City (1971), Amsterdam (1973), Jerusalem (1975), Helsinki (1977), Ottawa (1979), Paris (1981), Caracas (1983), Vienna (1985), Brussels (1989) and Hamburg (1991). The next four congresses are planned as follows: Montreal (1993), Venice (1995), Adelaide, Australia (1997) and the Netherlands (1999). It will hopefully then be the turn of the Far East – possibly China or Taiwan.

The IASP, to use the normal abbreviation of the association, brings together suicide researchers, clinicians, interdisciplinary workers of various categories and volunteers, for example from telephone services, from around the world. The latest treatments and preventive measures at national and international level are discussed. The nationally elected representatives meet to discuss their problems with a mutual exchange of experiences. The organisation has seen it as its task to promote suicide prevention measures in those parts of the world where suicide prevention is considered to need special strengthening.

A main topic is selected for each congress. At the Brussels congress this was suicide in the young and biological factors in suicide and in Hamburg the topic was suicide in the elderly. A Stengel Prize was set up at the Helsinki congress, to be awarded at each congress to the young researcher(s) who has or have produced the best research in the field of suicidology.

In 1965 the Association founded its own newsletter, *VITA*, which existed until 1979. Since 1980 the specialist journal of the Association has been *CRISIS*, edited by Battegay and since 1991 by Kerkhof and Clark. The journal is published four times per year. In addition, an IASP Newsletter is sent to all members, again four times per year. Individual national associations also publish their own journals. The most influential is the journal of the American association, *Suicide and Life-Threatening Behavior*. The former West Germany acquired its own in 1974, *Suizidprophylaxe. Theorie und Praxis*. The most recent national journal is the Italian one, *Giornale Italiano di Suicidologia*, established in 1991. The secretariat of the IASP is in Vienna (Central Administrative Office, Severingasse 9, A-1090 Vienna, Austria). Individual member dues (1992) are US $50, the same for member associations.

Although the IASP has also seen it as its task to initiate and promote research in suicidology, it gradually became clear that it would be desirable to have a separate organisation for this purpose. The International Academy for Suicide Research was founded in 1990, on the initiative of René Diekstra from the Netherlands. This academy, whose members have to be elected members from the international research forum, is to have special responsibility for stimulating and coordinating suicide research of high quality. A new journal has been started under the auspices of the Academy – *The Archives of Suicide Research*. IASP co-operates closely with this organisation and with the International Federation of Telephonic Emergency Services IFOTES.

IASP is a member of and cooperates closely with the WHO and the World Federation of Mental Health. The IASP in co-operation with the WHO is in the process of producing a WHO publication on suicide prevention strategies in developing countries. The WHO has also asked the IASP, in co-operation with the International Academy for Suicide Research, to draw up a position paper on the definition and classification of suicidal acts, for possible use as a supplement to the new diagnosis manual in ICD-10 (10th edition of the international classification system, WHO 1991).

Finally it must be mentioned that European research conferences are held every other year – in Bologna in 1990 and Odense in 1992.

International cooperation in suicidology is obviously of the greatest importance for promoting suicide prevention work around the world.

Research

This is a key task in connection with treatment and prevention. Intensive research work underlies most of the advances made in medicine, including suicidology. Much of what we know with regard to suicide and attempted suicide we know because of the intensive research that has been carried out, particularly over the past three to four decades, and under the international measures that have been discussed.

Only a limited number of countries supply suicide statistics. It is probable that no national registers are maintained in any country with regard to attempted suicide. There are no epidemiological studies showing how often suicide attempts which did not lead to admissions to hospitals or institutions are made. It is felt that they occur often. It would be of particular interest to know how this group gets on compared with those who are admitted. Studies employing epidemiological methods could make valuable contributions. The World Health Organisation has now started a programme to analyse attempted suicide in a number of countries, and has included two centres in Norway (Sør-Trøndelag and Østfold). The clinical research tasks are obviously great and many. The effectiveness of the methods of treatment must be made the subject of in-depth analyses. Risk factors must be better elucidated. The subsequent fate of those who attempt suicide must be analysed. Norway can presumably continue to make important contributions to suicide research in the future. It ought to be able to contribute significant results on the incidence of suicide in groups of the population, in groups of patients with mental illnesses and in groups with physical ailments. The incidence of suicide for example in cancer patients and in drug and alcohol abusers could also be surveyed more thoroughly. Several research programmes are in progress in Norway, and there is significant cooperation with the rest of Scandinavia and with international research. Examples of Norwegian and Nordic research have been quoted at several places in this book.

Tertiary prevention

By this I mean measures which are concerned with treatment and which can prevent the person threatened by suicide from committing suicide. This has been discussed in depth elsewhere in the book. However, it must be pointed out that treatment in the institutions suffers from the fact that suicide theory is not being given sufficient space in syllabuses, either in medical studies, psychology studies, nursing studies or among staff working in psychiatric institutions. There is a need for more extensive teaching, both at the theoretical level and at the level of supervision in the ward. But there is also a need for frequent instruction and regularly repeated instruction. It is my hope that this book can provide a basis for such instruction in institutions, health and social centres, and in further training and advanced training courses both in Norway and elsewhere in the world.

Suicide and the media

It has been known for a long time that suicide is 'infectious'. If there has been a case of suicide in a village, in a family or in a hospital ward, people have always been on their guard to make sure that the next one is not around the corner. It is also known that there are consequences when a great deal of attention is focused on suicide which is presented in a dramatic fashion. When Goethe's *Werter's Leiden* became popular and captured minds in Europe, many suicides followed in its wake. It was not until the end of the 1960s and during the 1970s and 1980s that more scientific research was conducted on this topic.

Much of this research has come from the USA, particularly from D. P. Phillips, a professor of sociology (1977, 1989; Phillips & Carstensen, 1986). In 1974 he studied the monthly variation in suicide in the USA before and after publicised suicides in the newspapers (all suicides which were presented in a more or less sensationalist way). The basis was the presentation of a suicide in the New York Times. He examined publicised suicide stories in American newspapers and looked at how the suicide rate behaved in the various areas where readers of the relevant newspapers were located. He was able to show clearly that material published in the first half of the month led to an increase in suicide in the area in the relevant month, whilst publication in the second half of the month led to more of an increase in the month after. The increase takes place in the geographical area where the suicide story received most publicity. Phillips was then thinking that it was merely a triggering cause in people who were in any case on the verge of committing suicide, and he therefore expected that the suicide rate would fall again afterwards. However, this fall did not occur. He tried out various hypotheses to explain the increase, and the best explanation he could come up with for the findings was that the somewhat sensationalist suicide stories act as a trigger mechanism to induce suicide, probably due to imitation. It was also found that in the USA an increase in suicide rate occurred when famous people or 'celebrities' committed suicide, such as Marilyn Monroe. Phillips (1979) has also shown that the number of road accidents increases, particularly accidents in which the driver was alone in the car. He was also able to show that in fatal accidents in the period immediately following a publicised suicide story in which only the driver was present, the drivers in the accident were rather similar to the person described in the story. His interpretation of this phenomenon is that suicide stories act as a trigger mechanism in increasing and inducing suicide, and some of these suicides are disguised as road accidents.

There has been some controversy over these findings in the scientific community, since the methodology is difficult in this area. But Phillips & Carstensen (1986) also described an increase in the suicide rate after television programmes depicting dramatic suicide events. Both Phillips and a British research group (Platt, 1987) have shown that soap operas in which a suicide attempt is made by a female character lead to an increase in the suicide rate precisely in women of the same age, who in many ways could be imagined as identifying themselves with the character.

However, no systematic research apart from the American studies had been carried out in this area before the psychologist Schmidtke and the psychiatrist Häfner in 1986 published a study entitled 'Die Vermittlung von Selbstmordmotivation und Selbstmordhandlung durch fiktive Modelle. Die Folgen der Fernsehserie Tod eines Schülers' ('The mediation of suicidal motivation and suicidal action through fictional models. The consequences of the television series Death of a Schoolboy'). They described a kind of *Werter effect* for this six-part television series which was broadcast in West Germany in 1981 under the title 'Death of a

Schoolboy'. The outcome of the suicidal act was repeated at the start of every episode, and the start of the suicidal act was shown in episodes two to six. The series was broadcast again in 1982. Schmidtke and Häfner used this natural 'experiment' as the basis for their research. The six episodes were broadcast for the first time in January and February 1981, with repeats in October and November 1982.

The student committed suicide by throwing himself in front of a train. The central office of statistics in West Germany does not list railway accidents separately, and the researchers therefore had to collect data themselves on suicide in relation to sex and age, railway accidents and the date of the suicidal act. Data was collected from all the German states. The student was 19-years-old. The researchers therefore focused on the group of young people aged between 15 and 29 who could be imagined as identifying most with this student. When they compared the period of the first transmission plus the following two weeks with the same period in the control period which was the years prior to that time, they found a clear increase in suicide rate for young people in this age group. The same trend was found when the period which stretched beyond two weeks, up to five weeks after the last episode, was studied. Figure 23.1 clearly demonstrating the peak is shown below.

Compared with the control years, there was an 86% increase for men in the period during which the TV programme was transmitted, plus five weeks after the last episode. In the case of women, there was an increase of 75%. When the authors looked at the 15 to 19 age group, those who were approximately the same age as the student, they found that the increase was greatest in this youngest group, and in this group 21 suicides were found compared with the expected 7.6 for the control years.

Corresponding results were found for the second run of the TV programme, in 1982. The number of male suicides increased by 54% at that time, and the increase was also greatest in the 15 to 20 age group.

The researchers were thus able to show clearly that an increase in the suicide rate occurred in connection with the transmitted television programmes, and that this increase was most marked in the same age group as the one the suicide in question was in, and that the increase applied in particular to the method the suicide in question had used. These findings strongly support Phillips' findings on the imitation effect, which apply particularly to people who are in a corresponding situation or age group. Whilst the American findings indicated that the increase

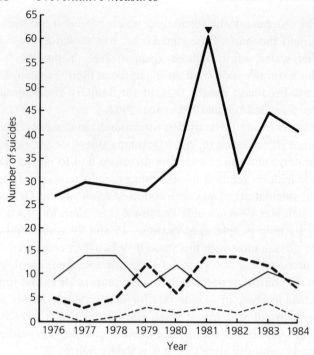

Figure 23.1. Suicide in the 1–20 age group during and after the first period of broadcasting (observation period 18 January 10 p.m. + 70 days; thick solid line men, thick broken line women) and in the control period (1 to 18 January 8 a.m.; solid line men, broken line women)

only takes place over a relatively short period afterwards, the German study showed that the increase continues for at least the first five weeks. Häfner and Schmidtke have also considered the possibility that these were marginal people who would have committed suicide anyway, and that the total number of suicides would even itself out on a yearly basis. However, this was not the case. No cases corresponding to this occurred afterwards. The authors therefore considered that transmitting such programmes leads to a direct increase in the suicide rate among those who identify with the person committing suicide shown in the programme.

As the situation is now, we must anticipate that films and television programmes where the main character, with whom people identify, commits suicide, can have an 'infective' effect on people in corresponding age groups and situations. We must anticipate that corresponding effects can also occur in connection with radio programmes and newspaper reports, where the reports dwell on the dramatic aspects of the act and causal factors behind it. Norwegians are spared the press coverage of suicide familiar in many other countries. In a number of countries cases of suicide are publicised with the full name, a description of the method used and also the life-story behind the suicide. It may be assumed that reports of this kind can induce suicide in people who identify with the person the report relates to. We must hope that the discretion which has been shown in the Norwegian press will continue. Those responsible for programmes on television and radio have good reason to pay attention to the imitation effect shown by research, as described here.

These phenomena have implication for the prevention. From Vienna, Etzersdorfer *et al.* (1992) have reported that since its opening in 1978, the Viennese subway has been used as a place for committing suicide. Since 1984 there has been a sharp increase in its use because of the dramatic reports on these suicides in the major Austrian newspapers. In 1987 the Austrian Association for Suicide Prevention created media guidelines and requested the press to follow them. The quality in the reporting on suicide was markedly improved. At the same time the number of suicides in the subway rapidly decreased. The Vienna experience supports the hypothesis that press reports of suicide may trigger yet further suicides.

A Norwegian study (Riaunet *et al.*, 1991) on mass media reports of suicide and suicide attempts and the rate of suicide did not give any conclusive results. This may be due to the restrictions the main media in Norway has placed upon itself for the publishing of suicides.

The discussion of suicide and the mass media would not be correct if we stopped here. The mass media without doubt have an important mission to perform with regard to suicide prevention. This mission applies primarily to educational and information activity. As has been pointed out on several occasions in this book, it is of the greatest importance for the prevention of suicide for taboos to be broken down, and for knowledge of suicide in the population to be increased. All sober and sound educational and information activity is therefore of value in preventing suicide if it can generalise the problem of suicide and make people more understanding of those who attempt to take their own lives or have done so, and can lead to a less prejudicial attitude. People will then dare to talk to someone who has suicidal thoughts or has carried out such acts and understand that this is a person in distress and difficulty who is in need of human contact. As relations, friends, neighbours or workmates, everyone can act as an understanding fellow-being who can help and offer support, and perhaps directly prevent suicide by doing so. Our attitudes towards people who are facing suicidal problems can be greatly influenced by the media. The mass media are therefore partners with which to cooperate in the battle to prevent suicide.

24

Suicide prevention measures in the present-day perspective. Experience of national programmes – World Health Organization strategy

The WHO, Regional Office for Europe, considered the European situation to be a matter of great concern, and therefore arranged a working meeting from 25 to 28 September 1989 at Szeged in Hungary, under the title 'Consultation on Strategies for Reducing Suicidal Behaviour in the European Region'. The WHO has set a number of targets in the European strategy for health for all in the year 2000. Target no. 12 in this strategy is to reduce the suicide rate in European countries. It is pointed out by the WHO that in Europe around 135,000 people take their own lives every year. The trend has been for this figure to rise steadily, and in virtually all European countries. The trend is also for the increase to be greatest in the countries that previously have had a relatively low suicide rate, and in the youngest age groups and to some extent in the oldest age group. The increase has been greatest in the southern and central western areas of Europe, and in the Nordic countries the increase has been sharpest in Norway. The WHO, Regional Office for Europe has had a working group since 1981 to study the changing pattern of suicidal behaviour in Europe. In 1984 the thirty-two member states of the European region of the WHO adopted 38 targets for improving health for all in the year 2000. Target no. 12, as mentioned above, was to reduce the suicide rate. Projects were launched in 12 countries with a view to studies on suicide attempts in order to analyse the population which attempts suicide, and it is planned that this work will be concluded by 1993.

The working meeting in Szeged, Hungary, was arranged as an element in the attainment of the target set. The national programmes in the countries which have so far developed their own suicide prevention programmes were examined at this meeting. It appears that Finland has gone furthest in meeting these targets. There is an ambitious programme here to reduce the suicide rate by 20% by 1995. A strong commitment has been made to research and to local schemes. A central group has been set up to plan and implement this research, which is being directed by a research professor specific to this area – Jouko Lönnqvist of Helsinki. The intention is to analyse each individual suicide very precisely in the various counties of Finland and to have decentralised participation from, for example the police, experts in forensic medicine and researchers, and to ensure co-operation between the sectors. The initiative for the Finnish project came from Finnish research communities, but great emphasis has been put on decentralised participation. The precise analysis of the material is being carried out on the 1,400 or so suicides which took place in Finland between 1 April 1987 and 31 March 1988. There is specialist expertise in this analytical work in each individual county. Altogether around 300 people are taking part in the preliminary studies, which will be followed by preventive programmes as the expertise is built up.

In Sweden there has been major research in the field of suicide by such people as H.G. Dahlgren (1945), Ulf Otto (1971), Ruth Ettlinger (1975) and Jan Beskow (1979). Earlier in this book I looked at the statement presented by the Care Programme Committee of the Swedish National Board of Health and Welfare on suicide from 1983, with guidelines for programmes at regional, hospital and clinical levels, including models for the assessment of suicide risk. The Swedish Board of Health and Welfare in its 1985 report also issued guidelines for suicide prevention within the psychiatric treatment apparatus. We have also previously given information from this report. Since 1984 the Office of Psychiatry in the Swedish Directorate of Health has had a part-time consultant in suicidology. Guidelines for suicide prevention in the medical treatment apparatus are under preparation. Special training programmes have been put into effect in psychiatry courses with suicidology as a key topic. The Swedish Psychiatry Association held a three-day course on suicidology for all personnel in psychiatry in 1983.

Considerable research activity is taking place in Sweden, chiefly in the field of biological psychiatry, under the direction of Marie Åsberg of the Karolinska Hospital in Stockholm, and in the psychological and social area by Jan Beskow in Gothenburg. In the biological field, substantial research is also being carried out by Professor Lil Träskman and co-workers at the Suicide Research Center in Lund. Some counties have also established their own suicide prevention measures. A suicide prevention programme was under way in the county of Skaraborg between 1979 and 1986 under the direction of Jan Beskow. A similar programme has been running in the county of Västerbotten since 1979 under the direction of Professor Lars Jacobsson. A depression and suicide prevention programme has also been in progress on Gotland since 1982. A special crisis centre for suicidal patients has been set up at Huddinge Hospital in Stockholm where Wolk Wasserman (1986, 1988) has made important contributions to research. The aim in Sweden is to bring about closer cooperation between the researchers in the area of the suicide problem, increase research, publish a yearbook concerned with suicidology, establish a special suicide prevention centre with responsibility for epidemiological analysis and local programmes, and finally to assess the suicide prevention programmes which have been carried out.

An educational programme for general practitioners was introduced on the Swedish island of Gotland, with the aim of increasing the knowledge among the practitioners about depression, its diagnosis and treatment. The suicide rate dropped significantly during the year after the implementation of the programme (Rutz, von Knorring & Wålinder, 1989).

Considerable experience has also been gathered in the Netherlands, where suicide prevention programmes have been planned to a considerable extent. An overview is given below of what has been achieved (Diekstra, 1988).

Research and information have been put first. It is considered to be vital to obtain up-to-date, correct data on the rate of both suicide and attempted suicide, and the characteristics of the people involved. The collection of data is of particularly great importance. In addition, multidisciplinary research is planned in which risk factors are to be assessed in selected groups. Well-planned studies of programmes of treatment for those who attempt suicide and preventive programmes for risk groups must be carried out, including with control groups. It must also be analysed how the educational activity towards groups such as for example therapists and teachers, and towards the public should be conducted.

The next item on the programme is to improve services provided to those who attempt suicide. Here it is of the greatest importance to raise the level of competence for health-care workers within the various professions in the treatment of depression and attempted suicide. They must be trained to identify and treat people who are in high-risk groups. The teaching of those groups who should preferably be most specialised must be intensified. This applies not least to psychiatrists, psychotherapists, clinical psychologists, general practitioners, internal medicine specialists and social workers and nurses. It is of great importance that programmes of instruction in suicidology for these groups should be made compulsory. The training programmes must incorporate knowledge in fields such as for example epidemiology, pathology and risk factors, but must also contain elements of interviewing techniques, treatment, including family treatment and after-care, and the treatment of the bereaved when a suicide has been carried out. The departments of the mental health service (Community Mental Health Centres) in each area must be made responsible for the coordination of care and treatment for persons at risk of suicide and for the development both of treatment models and training programmes. It is recommended that there should be an acute ward in each hospital for the treatment of attempted suicide and that psychiatric and psychological expertise is attached to this, and that psychiatric treatment can also be offered. Provision must be made in the acute wards for the suicidal patients to be kept over a long period, including when the purely somatic treatment has been completed. Co-operation must be established between the acute ward in a hospital and the psychiatric treatment apparatus in the same area. Research programmes and treatment programmes must be established at the psychiatric hospitals, and greater emphasis must be put on giving the staff practice in dealing with suicidal patients. Training programmes of a systematic nature and regularly repeated are necessary, because groups of personnel are constantly being replaced.

Training and information for particular groups in the population are also necessary. Training programmes must be established for teachers and school advisers, and teachers must recognise the signs of serious depression and the risk of suicide among their pupils. A training programme of this kind must contain some training in suicidology in general, on signs of depression or other psychological disturbances, knowledge of how further referrals can be made and how the suggestion of suicidal behaviour should be met. Similar programmes of training should also be given to the police, since the police very often come into contact with suicidal people, either through threats or attempts, and because the police should also be contacted when suicide has been carried out. Guidelines for how police are to behave when called to a suicide must be clear, such as that they should wear civilian clothes, not leave the relatives alone until other members of the family or neighbours have arrived, get in touch with the family doctor and show some degree of discretion. They also have to be taught to take care of suicide notes, diaries, etc., which may be of significance in clarifying the causal factors.

It is also important to develop a telephone service, for example in the form set up by the Church, and to study the types of people who benefit from this type of service.

There should also be educational programmes for the general public, in the press and on television, discreet in nature but in which the phenomenon is generalised and people are taught to interpret signals of depression and suicidal attempts or acts. Special programmes should be set up for journalists.

Special groups need extra attention. This applies to the youngest age groups and the oldest, and people suffering from depression, psychoses and other psychiatric symptoms. Staff in nursing homes should also attend training programmes, and not least those who are involved in the treatment of alcoholics and drug abusers, since these groups are particularly at risk of suicide. The same applies to relations and close members of the family of people who have committed suicide, who also need special help. Active measures should be implemented to deal with them. Information should also be given to the bereaved in other ways, for example in the form of brochures and other types of printed matter which examine and offer advice on the special situation of the bereaved after a suicide.

There is a clear view, in the Finnish, Swedish and Dutch programmes, that suicide prevention work bears fruit and that systematic suicide prevention work is the only feasible route to follow in reducing the suicide rate.

It is recommended in all three countries that a central group should be set up at national level, consisting of researchers, politicians, health-care workers of various categories, educationalists, clergy, etc., who cooperate over the course of time to produce guidelines for suicide prevention measures within the individual country. It can be mentioned for example that the Dutch coordinating group consisted of 16 members who presented a major report on what suicide prevention measures should be carried out in the Netherlands.

A national suicide prevention programme is also being prepared in Norway. A group to draw up this programme was appointed in the spring of 1991, and preparation of the programme will be completed in 1992, under the auspices of the Norwegian Directorate of Health.

The WHO, on the basis of its meeting in Hungary, has made some recommendations which entail each member state being advised to set up a central coordinating body for suicide prevention work and implement suicide prevention measures in line with the recommendations of this body.

The WHO has viewed with concern the rising suicide rate, not least in the European countries. The Regional Office for Europe has therefore wanted to establish a strategy for ways of reversing the rising trend and achieving what is the WHO's target in this area – the present upward trend in the suicide rate and the incidence of attempted suicide must have been reversed by the year 2000. This is the background to the meeting referred to above at Szeged in Hungary, attended by 21 delegates from 10 countries. The author of this book took part as an adviser, and also in his capacity as President of the IASP. The conclusions and recommendations are as follows.

World Health Organization recommendations to European governments

The working group concluded that there was a great need to develop and improve coordinated national and multinational strategies for preventive work, chiefly along the following lines:

- Train the public, particularly the politicians, to be aware of social and individual factors which increase the risk of suicide and which can provide the basis for prevention programmes.
- Train health-care personnel of all categories in the subject of suicidology.
- Improve the function the health-care and social services have in detecting the risk of suicide and in dealing with individuals and groups who have a high risk of suicidal behaviour.
- Expand and improve the coordination, at both the national and international level, of suicide research with regard to epidemiological data and the measurement of the effects of prevention programmes.

When national and regional programmes are to be drawn up, it is necessary to be aware of the following: suicidal behaviour never exists in isolation, but is involved in a complex interrelationship of behavioural, emotional, interpersonal and social factors, which must each be looked at separately, at the individual level, at the family level and at the social level. Research and intervention programmes should therefore not be exclusively focused on suicidal behaviour, but on groups and behaviour which are known to be related, and which are often found simultaneously (such as, for example, alcohol and drug abuse, and mental disorders).

There is a lack of adequate data for measuring the effect of prevention programmes. There is statistical data on suicide in most countries, but there are very few countries which have national or regional data on suicide attempts. It is necessary to have these data if it is to be possible to measure the effect of preventative work.

There is also a lack of national and international standardisation of definitions and terminology, making comparisons between countries difficult. It will be important to produce standard definitions and guidelines for using them.

National programmes and strategies have been developed in countries such as Finland, Sweden and the Netherlands. The initiative for devising such programmes has usually come from research groups which have pointed to the suicide problem on a national basis, and who have in particular brought it to the attention of politicians and especially health policy-makers, but who have also made the public aware of it through the media. It is important to establish co-operation between research, universities and other institutions and health-care workers if national and local programmes are to be developed.

Contrary to what is expected, both by the public and by the politicians, those who are regarded as experts in suicide prevention work in many countries are unfortunately very inadequately trained with respect to suicidology. This lack of training among the professional health-care personnel is cause for great concern. Steps must therefore be taken to develop adequate training programmes in suicidology. Suicidology *must be a compulsory subject* in the training of all health-care workers, both psychiatric and other health-care workers.

Suicide prevention programmes must not only be targeted specifically at risk groups but also at attitudes among treating personnel and the public, because these attitudes can be of great significance to the identification of the danger of suicide and how such a danger is to be met and treated.

A logical consequence of these considerations is that the scope and assessment of suicide prevention programmes can be measured not just in terms of changes in the suicide rate and the incidence of suicide attempts but also in terms of what percentage of the total health-care budget is taken up by suicide prevention work. Suicide prevention work can also be measured by indicating the percentage of health-care workers who have received compulsory instruction in suicidology in their training, and in the number of health-care workers who are given instruction in suicidology annually and in the number of seminars and training programmes in suicidology that are given. It can also be measured in terms of the number of publications and the number of public programmes, for example on the radio, on television and in the press, which are intended to educate the public on suicidology. In addition, it can be measured in terms of the number of institutions, both psychiatric and other medical institutions, which have programmes for the after-care of patients who have been treated for attempted suicide.

As suicide occurs in all countries, international co-operation is essential, and institutions such as the WHO and the IASP must take a leading role in this international co-operation.

WHO recommendations

The working group wishes to make the following recommendations to the member states.

- Recognise and establish that the problem of suicide and attempted suicide must have a high priority in public health policy.
- Take the necessary steps to develop national programmes for the prevention of suicide, where necessary in conjunction with other preventative health programmes, such as programmes for the prevention of mental disorders in general, prevention of drug abuse and prevention of damage.
- Establish national coordinating committees consisting of health policy-makers, researchers, therapists and representatives of other relevant groups. These coordinating committees should preferably be appointed by, or be closely linked to, the central health management, directorate of health or department of health, or equivalent organisations.

The objective of such coordinating committees should be:

- To collect and disseminate information on suicidal behaviour, causes and measures for treatment and prevention.
- To promote the formation of sub-national, regional and local networks of health policy-makers, researchers, health-care workers and representatives of other groups in order to appoint corresponding groups in the local communities and promote the coordination of prevention programmes and the training of the public.
- To increase awareness among politicians, health policy-makers, health-care workers, the media and the public of the significance of the suicide problem, its causes and connection with other related

problems, such as alcohol and drug abuse, and discuss the options for preventative programmes.

- To promote the development and use of training programmes in suicidology for all relevant categories of health-care personnel, such as general practitioners, psychiatrists, other medical specialists, nurses, social workers and other personnel who come into contact with people, as for example the police, ambulance personnel, prison personnel, teachers and telephone service volunteers.
- To promote the coordination of research which takes place and encourage further research.
- To develop and promote the use of guidelines and programmes to improve the health service and social service which is given to suicidal persons and also to close relatives and to local groups around the suicidal individuals.

Appendix – Legal aspects

In the original Norwegian edition this section appeared as a chapter but as this translated edition is aimed at a more international readership it was felt, therefore, that it would be more useful as an appendix as it is not within the scope of this book to cover all the international legal aspects on suicide.

International legislation

Legislation on both attempted suicide and suicide has followed the social trends which have prevailed at different times according to the view taken of suicide, not least that of the religious views. Reference was made in chapter 2 to the many synods which passed resolutions concerning suicide.

In England it is known for certain that attempting suicide was branded a crime from 1745. This law was not repealed until 1961. The author of this book practised in psychiatric hospitals in England while these statutory provisions were still in force (1956). The law created great problems in the treatment of patients who had attempted suicide, since they risked being brought before a court of law if someone had reported them for the attempted suicide before they were admitted to hospital. An important task for doctors was therefore to issue declarations that it was illness that had driven them to attempt suicide. A good certificate to this effect could save the person concerned from prosecution. The last person to be convicted for attempted suicide in England was sentenced to two years imprisonment. This was as recently as 1960. The person concerned was a prisoner who had tried to take his own life in his cell, and was punished by a further two years in prison.

Attempted suicide is still punishable in some countries, principally those countries which have in the past been under British rule, such as Canada and in particular India. It is a punishable offence to assist a person to commit suicide in most countries, including Norway.

Norwegian legislation

As mentioned in chapter 2, suicide was considered to be a form of dishonourable killing under Norwegian law. In the Norwegian statute-book of 1687, Christian V's Norwegian Law, which was also applicable in Iceland and on the Faeroes, it was stipulated that a person who took his own life was not to be buried in a church or churchyard unless he had taken his own life in sickness or rage. With regard to the position of the priest in relation to corpses, it was laid down that 'They must not throw earth on or hold a funeral service over someone who for his misdeed has been executed or has murdered himself by his own will.'

It was not just the 'body and soul' of the person who committed suicide that was subject to punishment. The survivors were also affected in that the inheritance or fortune of the person who committed suicide were to fall to the King or what today would be called the Treasury. 'He who takes his own life has forfeited his allotment to his family and must not be buried either in a church or a churchyard unless he does so in sickness or rage.'

On the other hand, there was no punishment for attempted suicide in Christian V's Norwegian statute-book. The question of whether attempted suicide should be punishable was examined by the Penal Act Commission of 1828. The Penal Act Commission rejected punishment for attempted suicide on the logical grounds that any punishment could drive the person who made the attempt actually to commit suicide later.

The Penal Act of 1842 repealed the provision that the fortune of the person committing suicide should not fall to the family but to the State. The same law also repealed the provision that the person who committed the suicide could not be buried in consecrated soil. The prohibition on throwing earth onto the body was repealed by a law of 1897. The prohibition of funeral services for those who had committed suicide was lifted by a law of 1902. Since 1902, legislation has been restricted to imposing penalties for assisting suicide, as is the case in most countries.

There are special legal problems in relation to suicide and life assurance. Most insurance companies make special exclusions with regard to suicide. The following exclusion is usual in connection with life-assurance policies in Norway, 'If the insured dies in the first two years after the policy has been taken out or resumed, and the cause of death is suicide, the insurance is only valid where there are grounds for assuming that the policy was taken out without thought of suicide. If the policy becomes invalid, the company will repay the premiums without interest, provided the policy covers the risk of death.' However, it is the insurance company which has to prove that the insurance was taken out with a view to suicide, which is of course difficult. As far as I know, the law has not been applied in Norway.

The situation with regard to accident insurance is different, since suicide has usually been excluded from the term accident.

Bibliography

Presented here are the major references since 1980 on suicide and attempted suicide together with the more classical older works. (Where possible translations of titles have been given.) A review of the literature before 1970 can be found in Retterstøl (1970) *Selvmord* [Suicide] and a review of the literature for the period 1970–78 can be found in Retterstøl (1978) *Selvmord, død og sorg* [Suicide, death and berievement] both published by Universitetsforlaget, Oslo.

Achté, K. A. & Lönnqvist, J. (1975). Suicide in Finnish culture. In *Suicide in different cultures*, ed. N. L. Farberow. Baltimore: University Press.

Achté, K. & Vikkula J. (1984). SOS-Service – A suicide prevention center. In *Ut av sinnets labyrinter*, ed. A. A. Dahl & A. Sund, pp. 56–8. Oslo: Universitets-forlaget.

Achté, K., Aalberg, V. & Lönnqvist, J. (Ed.) (1980). *Psychopathology of Depression*. Psychiatria Fennica Supplementum.

Allardt, E. (1975). *Att ha, att älska, att vara. Välfärd i Norden.* Lund: Argos.

Alnæs, R. (1990). Suicid under psykiatrisk behandling. [Suicide under psychiatric treatment.] *Nord. Psykiatr. Tidsskr.*, **44**, 41–9.

Arner, O. (1970). *Dødsulykker blant sjømenn.* [Accidental deaths among sailors.] Oslo: Universitetsforlaget.

American Psychiatric Association (1987). *Diagnostic and statistical manual of mental disorders*, 3rd revised edtn. DMS-III.R. Washington: American Psychiatric Association.

Arngrim, T. (1975). *Attempted suicide. Etiology and long term prognosis.* Odense: Odense University Press.

Banki, C. M., Arato, M., Papp, Z. & Kurcz, M. (1984). Biochemical markers in suicidal patients. Investigations with cerebrospinal fluid, amine metabolites and neuroendocrine tests. *J. Affective Disord.*, **6**, 341–50.

Banki, C. M. *et al.* (1985). Cerebrospinal fluid magnesium and calcium related to amine metabolites, diagnosis, and suicide attempts. *Biol. Psychiatry*, **20**, 163–71.

Beskow, J. (1979). Suicide and mental disorder in Swedish men. *Acta Psyciatr. Scand. Supp.*, **227**. Copenhagen: Munksgaard.

243

244   *Bibliography*

Beskow, J. (1987). The prevention of suicide while in psychiatric care. *Acta Psychiatr. Scand. Suppl.*, **336**(76), 66–75.

Beskow, J. (1989). *Country report: Sweden.* Consultation on Strategies for Reducing Suicidal Behaviours in the European Region, Szeged, Hungary 25–28 September.

Bille-Brahe, U. (1987). A pilot study of the level of integration in Norway and Denmark. *Acta Psychiatr. Scand. Suppl.*, **336**, 45–62.

Bille-Brahe, U. *et al.* (1987). *Selvmord og selvmordsforsøg.* [Suicide and attempted suicide.] Copenhagen: Hans Reitzels Forlag.

Bjerke, T. (1990). Selvmordsatferd blant studenter og andre grupper unge voksne. [Suicide among students and other groups of young people.] *Tidsskr. Nor. Psykologforen*, **27**, 438–46.

Bjerke, T. (1991). *Selvmord og selvmordsforsøk blant unge.* [Suicide and attempted suicide among the young.] Trondheim: Tapit.

Bjerke, T. & Stiles, T. C. (Eds.) (1991). *Suicide attempts in the Nordic countries.* Trondheim: Tapir.

Bjerk, T., Rygnestad, T. & Stiles, T. C. (1991). Epidemiological and clinical aspects of parasuicide in the county of Sør-Trøndelag, Norway. In *Suicide attempts in the Nordic countries*, ed. T. Bjerke, & T. C. Stiles. Trondheim: Tapir.

Bowlby, J. (1969) *Attachment and loss.* New York: Basic Books.

Bratfos, O. (1971) Attempted suicide. A comparative study of patients who have attempted suicide and pychiatric patients in general. *Acta Psychiatr. Scand.*, **47**, 38–56.

Bravermann, E. R. & Pfeiffer, C. C. (1981). Suicide and biochemistry. *Biol. Psychiatry*, **20**, 123–24 (editorial).

Bämayr, A. (1983). *Über den Selbstmord von 119 Ärzten, Ärztinnen, Zahnärzten und Zahnärztinnen in Oberbayern von* 1963 *bis* 1978. Munich Max-Planck-Institut für Psychiatrie.

Central Bureau of Statistics of Norway (1987). *Norwegian official statistics. Health statistics* 1987. Oslo.

Crepet, P., Caracciolo, S., Casoli, R., Fabri, D., Grassi, G., Tomelli, A. & Jorus, A. (1990). Suicidal behaviour in Emilia Romagna Region: preliminary results from 1988–1990 monitoring of parasuicide. In *Suicidal behaviour and risk factors*, ed. G. Ferrari, M. Bellini, & P. Crepet. 201–5. Bologna: Monduzzi.

Dahlgren, K. G. (1945). *On suicide and attempted suicide.* Lund: Lindstedts Univ. Bokhandel.

Dahlgren, K. G. (1977). Attempted suicide – 35 years afterward. *Suicide Life Threat. Behav.*, **7**, 75–9.

Dalgard, O. S. (1966). Mortalitet ved funksjonelle psykoser. *Nord. Med.*, **75**, 680–84.

De Leo, D., Degli Stefani, M., Dal Cin, B., Cadamuro, M., Caneva, A. & Banon, D. (1990). The problems of suicidal repetition: a study of data 1980–1988. In *Suicidal behaviour and risk factors*,, ed. G. Ferrari, M. Bellini, & P. Crepet. Bologna: Monduzzi.

De Leo, D. & Ormskerk, S. C. R. (1991). Suicide in the elderly: general characteristics. *Crisis*, **12**, 3–17.

Diekstra, R. F. W. (1988). Toward a comprehensive strategy for the prevention of suicidal behaviour: a summary of recommendations of national task forces. *Crisis*, **9**, 119–29.

Diekstra, R. F. W. (1989a). *Country report: Netherlands.* Consultation on

Strategies for Reducing Suicidal Behaviours in the European Region, Szeged, Hungary, 25–28 September.

Diekstra, R. F. W. (1989b). Suicidal behaviour in adolescents and young adults: the international picture. *Crisis*, **10**, 16–35.

Directory of Suicide Prevention Facilities (1967). *Bull. Suicidology*, **1**, 14–18.

Directory of Suicide Prevention Facilities (1969). *Bull. Suicidology*, **5**, 47–58.

Dorpat, L., Anderson, W. F. & Ripley, H. R. (1968). The relationship of physical illness to suicide. In *Suicidal behavioral diagnosis and management*, ed. H. P. L. Resnik. Boston: Little, Brown & Co.

Durkheim, E. (1912). *Le suicide*. Paris: Librairie Felix Alcan.

Durkheim, E. (1952). *Suicide*. London: Routledge, Kegan & Paul. (Transl.)

Eitinger, L., Retterstøl, N. & Malt, U. (1984). *Psykoser*. [Psychoses.] Oslo: Universitetsforlaget.

Eitinger, L. & Retterstøl, N. (1990). *Rettspsykiatri*. [Forensic psychiatry.] Oslo: Universitetsforlaget.

Eitinger, L., Retterstøl, N. & Dahl, A. A. (in cooperation with Malt, U.) (1991). *Kriser og nevroser*. [Crises and neuroses.] Oslo: Universitetsforlaget.

Ekeberg, Ø. (1992). Nasjonalt program for selvmordsforebyggende arbeid. [National programme for suicide prevention.] Oslo: Ministry of Health and Social Affairs.

Ekeberg, Ø., Ellingsen, Ø., & Jacobsen, D. (1991). Suicide and other causes of death in a five-year follow-up period of patients treated for self-poisoning in Oslo. *Acta. Psychiatr. Scand.*, **83**, 432–7.

Ekeberg, Ø., Frederichsen P. & Holan, L. (1985). Selvmordsstatistikkens pålitelighet i Norge. [Accurate suicide statistics for Norway.] *Tidsskr. Nor. Lægeforen*, **105**, 123–27.

Ekeberg, Ø. et al. (1988). Effects of deregistration of drugs and prescription recommendations on the pattern of selfpoisoning. In *Current issues of suicidology*, ed. H.-J. Möller & R. Welz, pp. 443–5. Berlin: Springer.

Etlinger, R. W. (1975). Evaluation of suicide prevention after attempted suicide. *Acta Psychiatr. Scand. Suppl.*, **260**, Copenhagen: Munksgaard.

Etzersdorfer, E., Sonneck, G. & Nagel-Kuess, S. (1992). Newspaper reports and suicide. *N. Engl. J. Med.*, **321**, 502–3.

Farber, M. (1968). *Theory of suicide*. Funk & Wagnalls.

Farberow, N. L. (Ed.) (1975). *Suicide in different cultures*. Baltimore: University Press.

Farberow, N. L. (1975). Cultural history of suicide (pp. 77–94). In *Suicide in different cultures*, ed. N. L. Farberow. Baltimore: University Press.

Farberow, N. L. (Ed.) (1980). *The many faces of suicide. Indirect self-destructive behavior*. New York: McGraw-Hill.

Faria, J. G. S. (1989). *The work of WHO for attaining target 12 of the European Strategy for Health for All by the Year* 2000. Consultation on Strategies for Reducing Suicidal Behaviour in the European Region, Szeged, Hungary 25–28 September.

Finzen, A. (1989). *Suizid-prophylaxe bei psychischen Störungen. Leitlinien für den therapeutischen Alltag*. Bonn: Psyciatrie-Verlag.

Fuchs, A., Gaspari, C. & Millendorfer, J. (1977). *Makropsychologische Untersuchung der Familie in Europa*. Studiengruppe für internationale Analysen, Berggasse 16, A-1090 Wien.

Garfinkel, B. D. & Golombek, H. (1983). Suicidal behaviour in adolescents. In *The adolescent and mood disturbances*, ed. B. D. Garfinkel & H. Golombek, pp. 189–217. New York: International University Press.

246   Bibliography

Gibbs, J. P. & Martin W. T. (1964). *Status integration and suicide. A sociological study.* Oregon: University of Oregon.
Giddenes, A. (Ed.) (1971). *The sociology of suicide. A selection of reading.* London: Frank Cass.
Gjertsen, F. (1987). *Selvmord i Norge.* [Suicide in Norway.] Hovedoppgave i sosiologi. Institutt for sosiologi, University of Oslo.
Gould, M. S. & Shaffer, D. (1989). The impact of suicide in television movies. In *Suicide and its prevention. The role of attitude and imitation*, ed. R. F. W. Diekstra *et al.*, pp. 331–40. Leiden: Brill.
Grove, O. & Lynge, J. (1979). Suicide and attempts in Greenland. *Acta Psychiatr. Scand.*, **60**, 375–91.
Hamburg, D. (1989). Preparing for life: the critical transition of adolescence. *Crisis*, **10**, 4–15.
Hammerlin, Y. (1992). Selvmord i norske fengsler, 1956–okt. 1991. [Suicide in Norwegian prisons 1956 to Oct. 1991.] *KRUS-Rapport*, Nr.1, Oslo.
Hammerlin, Y. & Enerstvedt, R. T. (1988). *Selvmord.* [Suicide.] Oslo: Falken Forlag.
Hawton, K. & Catalan, J. (1987). *Attempted suicide. A practical guide to its nature and managements.* Oxford: Oxford Medical Publications.
Hawton, K. & Fagg, J. (1988). Suicide and other causes of death, following attempted suicide. *Br. J. Psychiatry*, **152**, 359–66.
Helsedirektoratet [Ministry of Health.] (1987). *Helse for alle i Norge?* [Health for all in Norway?] Oslo: Kommuneforlaget.
Hendin, H. (1964). *Suicide and Scandinavia.* New York: Grune & Stratton.
Hendin, H. (1971). *Black Suicide.* New York: Harper & Row.
Hendin, H. (1978). Suicide: the psychosocial dimension. *Suicide Life Threat Behav.*, **8**, 99–117.
Hendin, H. (1982). *Suicide in America.* New York: Norton.
Hessø, R. (1977). Suicide in Norwegian, Finnish and Swedish psychiatric hospitals. *Arch. Psychiatr. Nervenkr.*, **224**, 119–27.
Hessø, R. (1987). Routines and practices in the registration of suicide in Scandinavia. *Acta Psychiatr. Scand. Suppl.* **336**, 17–21.
Hessø, R. & Retterstøl, N. (1975). Suicid i norske psykiatriske sykehus. [Suicide in Norwegian psychiatric hospitals.] *Tidsskr. Nor. Lægefor.*, **95**, 1571–4.
Hjortsjø, T. (1983). *Självmord i Stockholm. En epidemiologisk studie av 686 konsekutiva fall.* [Suicide in Stockholm. An epidemiological study of 686 cases.] Göteborg: Rapport, Nordiska Hälsovårdshögskola.
Hjortsjø, T. (1985a). Självmord i bildkonsten, del I. [Suicide in art.] *Draco pro Medico*, **26**, 8–13.
Hjortsjø, T. (1985b). Självmordsmotivet i västerländsk bildkonst. [Motives for suicide in western art.] *Tidsskr. Nor. Lægefor.*, **105**, 114–18.
Holdingen, P. C. (1979). Violent deaths among the young: Recent trends in suicide, homicide and accidents. *Am. J. Psychiatry*, **136**, 1144–47.
Hytten, K. & Weisæth L. (1989). Suicide among soldiers and young men in the Nordic countries 1977–1984. *Acta Psychiatr. Scand.*, **79**, 224–28.
Iga, M. & Tatai, K. (1975). Characteristics of suicides and attitudes towards suicide in Japan. In *Suicide in different cultures*, ed. N. L. Farberow, pp. 225–80. Baltimore: University Press.
Jónsdottir, G. (1977). Suicide in Iceland. In *Proceedings from IX Congress of Suicide Prevention and Crisis Intervention.* Helsinki.
Jónsdottir, G. & Sigurdsson, P. (1977). Diagnostik och registrering av självmord i Island. [Diagnosing and registering suicides in Iceland.] In *Proceedings from*

IX *Congress of Suicide Prevention and Crisis Intervention*, pp. 46–54. Helsinki.

Juel-Nielsen, N. (1984). Problemstillinger i nordisk selvmordsforskning. [Problems found within Nordic suicide research.] In *Ut av sinnets labyrinter*, ed. A. A. Dahl, & A. Sund, pp. 49–55. Oslo: Universitetsforlaget.

Juel-Nielsen, N. & Retterstøl, N. (1982). Selvmord i Norden. [Suicide in the Nordic countries.] *Nord Med* 57, pp. 265–66.

Juel-Nielsen, N. & Retterstøl, N. (1985). Selvmordsproblematikken i nordisk perspektiv. [The problem of suicide from a Nordic perspective.] *Medicinsk Årbog*. Copenhagen: Munksgaard.

Juel-Nielsen, N., Retterstøl, N. & Bille-Brahe, U. (1987). Suicide in Scandinavia. A report on the internordic research project. *Acta Psychiatr. Scand. Suppl.*, **336**.

Jørgensen, P. (Ed.) (1991). *Suicidal atferd i Norge*. [The suicidal process in Norway.] pp. 73–9. Oslo: Organon.

Jørstad, J. (1987). Some experience in psychotherapy with suicidal patients. *Acta Psychiatr. Scand. Supp.*, **336**, 76–81.

Kerkhof, A. J. F. M., Visser, A. & Diekstra, R. F. W. (1990). Strategie preventive nel compartemento suicidario degli anziani. In *Aspetti Clinici del Compartamento Suicidario*, ed. D. De Leo, Padova: Liviana editrice.

Kolmos, L. (1987). Suicide in Scandinavia: an epidemiological analysis. *Acta Psychiatr. Scand. Suppl.*, **336**, 11–16.

Kolmos, L. & Back, E. (1987). Sources of error in the registration of suicide. *Acta Psychiatr. Scand. Suppl.*, **336**, 22–44.

Kreitman, N. (1977). *Parasuicide*. London: Wiley.

Kreitman, N. (1980). The British anomaly: suicide, domestic gas and unemployment in the United Kingdom. In *Current issues of suicidology*, ed. H.-J. Möller, A. Schmidtke & R. Welz, pp. 364–71. Berlin: Springer.

Kreitman, N. (1988). Suicide, age and marital status. *Psychological Medicine*, **18**, 121–8.

Kreitman, N. & Casey, P. (1988). Repetition of parasuicide: an epidemiological and clinical study. *Brit. J. Psychiatry*, **153**, 792–800.

Krieger, G. (1970). Biochemical predictors of suicide. *Dis. Nerv. Syst.*, **31**, 479–82.

Kringlen, E. (1990). *Psykiatri*. [Psychiatry.] Oslo: Universitetsforlaget.

Lester, D. (1972). *Why people kill themselves: a summary of research findings on suicidal behaviour*. Springfield: Thomas.

Lester, D. (1974). Effect of suicide prevention centers on suicide rates in the United States. *Health Services Reports*, **89**, 37–9.

Lester, D. (1990). The effect of the detoxification of domestic gas in Switzerland on the suicide rate. *Acta Psychiatr. Scand.*, **82**, 383–4.

Lester, D. & Murel, M. (1982). The preventive effect of strict gun control laws on suicide and homicide. *Suicide Life Threat. Behav.* **12**, 131–40.

Linder, A. & Wang, A. G. (1988). Suicides among psychiatric patients in Funen, Denmark. In *Current issues of suicidology*, ed. H.-J. Möller, & R. Welz, pp. 70–74. Berlin: Springer.

Litman, R. E. (1972). Experiences in a Suicide Prevention Center. In *Suicide and attempted suicide*. Scandia International Symposia. Stockholm: Nordiska Bokhandelns Förlag.

Lynge, I. (1981). Suicide in Greenland. *Nordic Council for Artic Medical Research. Report* 27, pp. 88–92. Oulu.

Lönnqvist, J. (1977). *Suicide in Helsinki*. Helsinki: Monographs of Psychiatria Fennica.

Lönnqvist, J. (1989). *Country report: Finland*. Consultation on Strategies for Reducing Suicidal Behaviours in the European Region, Szeged, Hungary, 25–28 September.

Marzuk, P. M., Leon, A. C., Tardiff, K., Morgan, E. B., Stajic, M. & Mann, J. J. (1992). The effect of access to lethal methods of injury on suicide rates. *Arch. Gen. Psychiatry*, **49**, 451–8.

Mehlum, L. (1991). Selvmordsforsøk blant norske soldater. En retrospektiv undersøkelse. [Attempted suicide among Norwegian soldiers. A retrospective study.] *Tidsskr. Nor. Lægeforen.* **III**, 565–8.

Menninger, K. (1938). *Man against himself*. New York: Harvest Books, Harcourt, Brace & World.

Ministry of State, Department for Greenland Affairs (1989). *Yearbook for Greenland 1988*. Copenhagen.

Morild, I. (1988). *Selvpåførte forgiftninger og selvmord på Vestlandet 1978–1987*. [Self-poisoning and suicide in Vestlandet 1978–1987.] pp. 79–86. Oslo: Organon.

Murphy, G., Armstrong, J., Hemele, S., Fisher J. & Cleudewin, W. (1979). Suicide and alcoholism. *Arch. Gen. Psychiatry*, **36**, 65–9.

Murphy, G. & Robin, E. (1967). Social factors in suicide. *J. Am. Med. Ass.*, **199**, 303–8.

Murphy, G. & Wetzel, R. (1990). The lifetime risk of suicide in alcoholism. *Arch Gen. Psychiatry*, **47**, 383–92.

Murphy, G. E., Wetzel, R. D., Swallow, C. S. & McClure, J. N. Jr. (1969). Who calls the Suicide Prevention Center: a study of 55 persons calling on their own behalf. *Am. J. Psychiatry*, **126**, 314–22.

Naroll, R. (1983). *The Moral Order. An introduction to the Human Situation*. Sage, Beverly Hills.

Ninan, P. T. *et al.* (1984). CSF 5-hydroxyindolacetic acid levels in suicidal schizophrenic patients. *Amer. J. Psychiatry*, **141**, 566–69.

Nordic Medical Statistics Committee (1991). *Health statistics in the Nordic countries 1966–1991*. NOMESKO (Nordisk medicinal statistisk komité) 36, Copenhagen.

Noreik, K. (1966). Suicid ved funksjonelle psykoser. [Suicide and functional psychosis.] *Nord. Med.*, **75**, 158–61.

Noreik, K. (1971). Suicidalforsøk og suicid. [Attempted suicide and suicide.] *Tidsskr. Nor. Lægeforen*, **93**, 183–89.

Olafsen, O. M. (1983). Suicide among cancer patients in Norway. In *Depression and suicide*, ed. J. P. Soubrier, & J. Vedrinne, pp. 587–91. Paris: Pergamon Press.

Olafsen, O. M. (1984). Vurdering av suicidalfare. [Evaluation of the risk of suicide.] In *Ut av sinnets labyrinter*, ed. A. A. Dahl & A. Sund, pp. 59–66. Oslo: Universitetsforlaget.

Ostamo, A. & Lønnqvist, J. (1990). Parasuicide in Helsinki: a male problem. In *Suicidal behaviour and risk factors*, ed. S. Ferrari, M. Bellini & P. Crepet, pp. 185–8. Bologna: Monduzzi.

Ostamo, A. & Lønnqvist, J. (1991). Parasuicides in four catchment areas in Finland. In *Suicide attempts in the Nordic countries*, ed. T. Bjerke & T. C. Stiles. Trondheim: Tapir.

Otto, U. (1971). *Barns och ungdomars självmordshandlingar*. [Treatment for suicidal children and young people.] Akademisk avhandling. Stockholm: Karolinska institutet.

Ottosson, J. O. (1989). *Psykiatri.* Stockholm: Almqvist & Wiksell.

Perry, C. L. (1989). Teacher vs. peer-led intervention. *Crisis*, **10**, 52–61.

Pfeiffer, C. C. & D. Bacchi, (1975). Copper, zinc, manganese, niacin and pyridoxine in the schizophrenias. *J. Appl. Nutr.*, **27**, 9–39.

Phillips, D. P. (1977). Motor vehicle fatalities increase just after publicized suicide stories. *Science*, **195**, 1464–65.

Phillips, D. P. (1979). Suicide, motor vehicle fatalities and the mass media. Evidence toward a theory of suggestion. *Am. J. Sociology*, **79**, 1150–74.

Phillips, D. P. (1989). Recent advances in suicidology. The study of imitative suicide. In *Suicide and its prevention. The role of attitude and imitation*, ed. R. F. W. Diekstra, *et al.*, pp. 299–312. Leiden: Brill.

Phillips, D. P. & Carstensen, L. L. (1986). Clustering of teenage suicides after television news stories about suicide. *New Engl. J. Med.*, **315**, 685–89.

Platt, S. (1986). Suicide and parasuicide among further education students in Edinburgh. *Br. J. Psychiatry*, **150**, 183–8.

Platt, S. (1987). The aftermath of Angie's overdose: is soap (opera) damaging your health? *Brit. Med. J.*, **294**, 954–7.

Platt, S. (1989). Suicide trends in 24 European countries 1972–1984. In *Current issues of suicidology*, ed. H.-J. Möller, A. Schmidtke & R. Welz, pp. 3–13. Berlin: Springer.

Platt, S. (1990). Parasuicide in the European Region I Preliminary findings from WHO (EURO)-sponsered multicentre study. Paper presented at the *Third European Symposium on Suicidal Behaviour and Risk Factors. Bologna 25–28 September* 1990.

Prins, M. M. & Kerkhof, J. F. M. (1990). Epidemiology of suicide attempts in the Leiden area, the Netherlands. In *Suicidal behaviour and risk factors*, ed. G. Ferrari, M. Bellini & P. Crepet, pp. 195–200. Bologna: Monduzzi.

Pærregaard, G. (1963). *Selvmord og selvmordsforsøg i København.* [Suicide and attempted suicide.] Bind I, II og III. København.

Pöldinger, W. (1968). *Die Abschätzung der Suizidalität.* Huber, Bern.

Querejeta, I., Ballesteros, J., Salvador, J., Alonso, J., Blanco, L., Prieto, G., Zubia, C. & Korta, M. J. (1990). Parasuicide in a hospital-based catchment area. In *Suicidal behaviour and risk factors*, ed. G. Ferrari, M. Bellini & P. Crepet, pp. 207–10. Bologna: Monduzzi.

Rao, A. V. (1975). Suicide in India. In *Suicide in different cultures*, ed. N. L. Farberow. Baltimore: University Press.

Retterstøl, N. (1966). *Paranoid and paranoiac psychoses.* Springfield: Thomas.

Retterstøl, N. (1970). *Long-term prognosis after attempted suicide.* Universitetsforlaget, Oslo/Thomas, Springfield.

Retterstøl, N. (1975). Suicide in Norway. In *Suicide in different cultures*, ed. N. L. Farberow, pp. 77–94. Baltimore: University Press.

Retterstøl, N. (1987). *Stoffmisbruk.* 5 utg. [Drug abuse, 5th edition.] Oslo: Universitetsforlaget.

Retterstøl, N. (1988). Increasing suicide rate in Scandinavian psychiatric hospitals. In *Current issues of suicidology*, ed. H. J. Möller, A. Schmidtke & R. Welz, pp. 75–82. Berlin: Springer.

Retterstøl, N. (1989). Suicidal behaviour in Norway. Paper presented as WHO temporary adviser. Szeged, Hungary, 25–28 September.

Retterstøl, N. (1989). Norwegian data on death due to overdose of antidepressants. *Acta Psychiatr. Scand.*, **80**, Suppl. 354, 61–8.

Retterstøl, N. (1989). Selvmord – et økende problem i Norge. [Suicide – an increasing problem in Norway.] *Tidsskr. Nor. Lægeforen*, **109**, 3397–98.

Retterstøl, N., Ekeland, H. & Hessø, R. (1985). Selvmord hos unge. Utviklingen i Norden. Et 7-årsmateriale fra Oslo. [Suicide among the young. Development in Norway. A 7-year study from Oslo.] *Tidsskr. Nor. Lægeforen*, **105**, 119–22.

Retterstøl, N. & Opjordsmoen, S. (1990). Suicide in patients with delusional disorders. In *Psychiatry*, a world perspective, ed. C. N. Stefanis, A. D. Rabavilas & C. R. Soldatos, pp. 842–6. Amsterdam: Excerpta Medica.

Retterstøl, N. & Strype, B. (1973). Suicide attempts in Norway. A personal follow-up investigation. *Suicide Life Threat. Behav.*, **3**, 261–8.

Reynolds, D. K. & Farberow, N. L. (1977a). *Endangered hope. Experiences in psychiatric aftercare facilities.* Berkeley: University of California Press.

Reynolds, D. K. & Farberow, N. L. (1977b). *Suicide*, inside and out. Berkeley: University of California Press.

Riaunet, Å., Stiles, T. C., Rygnestad, T. & Bjerke, T. (1991). Mass media reports on suicide and suicide attempts and the rate of parasuicide. In *Suicide attempts in the Nordic countries*, ed. T. Bjerke & T. C. Stiles, pp. 152–62. Trondheim: Tapir.

Rich, C. L., Young, G., Fowler, R. C., Wagner, J. & Black, N. A. (1990). Guns and suicide: possible effects of some specific legislation. *Am. J. Psychiatry*, **147**, 342–6.

Richardson, R., Lowenstein, S. & Weissberg, M. (1989). Coping with the suicidal elderly: a physician's guide. *Geriatrics*, **44**, 43–7.

Riekl, T., Marchner, E., & Möller, H.-J. (1988). Influence of crisis intervention telephone services. (Crisis Hotlines) on the suicide rate in 25 German cities. In *Current issues of suicidology*, ed. H.-J. Möller, A. Schmidtke & R. Welz, pp. 431–6. Berlin: Springer.

Ringel, E. (1953). *Der Selbstmord*. Wien: Maudrich.

Ringel, E. (Ed.) (1969). *Selbstmordverhütung*. Bern: Huber.

Rüegsegger, P. (1963). Selbstmordversuche. *Psychiat Neurol. Basel.*, **146**, 81–104.

Rutz, W., von Knorring, L. & Wålinder, J. (1989). Frequency of suicide in Gotland after systematic postgraduate education of general practitioners. *Acta Psychiatr. Scand.*, **85**, 151–4.

Rygnestad, T. (1990). *Deliberate self-poisoning in Trondheim*. Trondheim: Tapir.

Sainsbury, P. (1955). *Suicide in London. An ecological study*. London: Chapman & Hall.

Sainsbury, P. (1963). Social and epidemiological aspects of suicide with special reference to the aged. In *Process of aging: social and psychological perspectives*, vol. 2, ed. R. H. Williams, C. Tibbiti & W. Donahue, pp. 151–76. New York: Atherton.

Sainsbury, P., Jenkins, J. & Levey, A. (1982). The social correlates of suicide in Europe. In *The suicide syndrome*, ed. R. Farmer & S. Hirsch. London: Croom Helm.

Salander-Renberg, E. & Jacobsson, L. (1991). Attempted suicide in Västerbotten county 1989. In *Suicide attempts in the Nordic countries*, ed. T. Bjerke & T. C. Stiles, pp. 69–78. Trondheim: Tapir.

Schmidtke, A. & Häfner, H. (1986). Die Vermittlung von Selbstmordmotivation und Selbstmordhandlung durch fiktive Modelle. Die Folgen der Fernsehserie – Tod eines Schülers, *Nervenarzt*, **57**, 502–10.

Schmidtke, A. & Häfner, H. (1988). Imitation effects after fictional television suicides. In *Current issues of suicidology*, ed. H.-J. Möller, A. Schmidtke & R. Welz, pp. 341–8. Berlin: Springer.

Schmidtke, A. & Häfner, H. (1989). Public attitudes towards and effects of the mass media on suicidal and deliberate selfharm behaviour. In *Suicide and its prevention. The role of attitude and imitation*, ed. R. F. W. Dickstra *et al.*, pp. 311–30. Leiden: Brill.

Schneider, P. B. (1954). *La tentative de suicide. Étude statistique, clinique, psychologique at catamnestique*. Neuchatel: Delachauz et Niestlé.

Schwartz, A. J. & Reifler, C. B. (1980). Suicide among American college and university students from 1970–71 through 1975–76. *J. Am. College Health Assoc.*, **21**, 205–10.

Seiden, R. H. (1984). Death in the west – a regional analysis of the youthful suicide rate. *Western J. Med.*, **140**, 969–73.

Shneidman, E. S. (Ed.) (1967). *Essays on Selfdestruction*. New York: Science House.

Shneidman, E. S. (1989). Approaches and commonalities of suicide. In *Suicide and its prevention. The role of attitude and imitation*, ed. R. F. W. Dickstra *et al.*, pp. 14–36. Leiden: Brill.

Sigurdsson, P. (1978). Dødsfrekvens av självmord i Island 1881–1976. [Rate of deaths from suicide in Iceland 1881–1976.] In *Nordisk symposium om forsking kring självmord*, Hanaholmen 27. – 29.11.1978, pp. 23–4. NOS-M.

Simon, W. (1989). Suicide among physicians: prevention and postvention. In *Suicide and its prevention. The role of attitude and imitation*, ed. R. F. W. Dickstra *et al.*, pp. 186–98. Leiden: Brill.

Skullberg, A. (1974). *Submersio og hypotermi*. Sandoz-informasjon fra forskning og praksis, vol. 4.

Sloan, J. H., Rivara, F. P., Reay, D. T., Ferris, J. A. J. & Kellerman, A. L. (1990). Firearm regulations and rates of suicide: a comparison of two metropolitan areas. *N. Eng. J. Med.*, **322**, 369–73.

Socialstyrelsen (1984). *Självmord inom den psykiatriska vården*. [Suicide in a psychiatric ward.] (Socialstyrelsens redovisar, 7.) Stockholm: Socialstyrelsen.

Socialstyrelsen. Vårdprogrammnämnden (1983). *Problemet självmord. Underlag till vårdprogram*. [The problem of suicide. The outline of a ward programme.] Utarb. av en arbetsgrupp under ledning av Jan Beskow. Socialstyrelsen, Stockholm.

Soubrier, J. P. & Vedrinne, J. (Ed.) (1983). *Depression and suicide*. Paris: Pergamon Press.

Stanley, M., Virgilio, J. & Gershon, S. (1982). Tritialed imipramine binding zites are deceased in the frontal cortex of suicides. *Science*, **216**, 1337–9.

Stanley, M. & Mann, J. J. (1984). Suicide and serotonin receptors. *Lancet*, **349**.

Statistisk Sentralbyrå (1984). *Helsestatistikk 1982*. NOS B 465. Oslo: Statistisk Sentralbyrå.

Stengel, E. (1967). *Suicide and attempted suicide*. London: Penguin Books.

Sundt, E. (1855). Om dødeligheten i Norge. Bidrag til kundskab til folkets kaar. [About mortality in Norway. Contribution to knowledge of the living condition for people.] Christiania: Malling.

Sundt, E. (1857). *Sædeligheds-Tilstanden i Norge*. Christiania: J. Chr. Abelsted.

Sundt, E. (1864). *Fortsatte Bidrag angaaende Sædeligheds-Tilstanden i Norge*. Christiania: Chr. Schibsted.

Tabachnick, H. (1967). The psychology of fatal accident. In *Essays on Selfdestruction*, ed. E. S. Shneidman, pp. 399–413. New York: Science House.

Tatai, K. & Tatai, K. (1991). Suicide in the elderly: a report from Japan. *Crisis*, **12**, 40–3.

Thorslund, J. (1989). Ungdomsselvmord i Grønland. [Suicide in youngsters in Greenland.] *Social Kritik*, **4**, 55–85.

Tuckman, J. & Youngman, W. F. (1963). Identifying suicide risk groups among attempted suicides. *Public Health Reports*, **78**, 763–6.

Tuckman, J. & Youngman, W. F. (1966). A scale for assessing suicide risk in attempted suicides. *J. Clin. Psychol.*, **24**, 17–19.

van Praag, H. M. (1983). CSF-5 HIAA and suicide in nondepressed schizophrenics. *Lancet*, **978**.

Varah, C. (1973). *The Samaritans in the '70s*. London: Constable.

Wang, A. G. (1989). *Suicidal behaviour in a low-incidence population – a study of the Faroe islanders*. Odense: Akademisk avhandling.

Wasserman, D. & Eklund, G. (1991). A study of socio-demographic factors in an unselected parasuicide population in Stockholm. In *Suicide attempts in Nordic countries*, ed. T. Bjerke & T. C. Stiles, pp. 79–90. Tondheim: Tapir.

Wedler, H. (1988). Catamnestic studies on patients who attempted suicide: an overview. In *Current issues of suicidology*, ed. H.-J. Möller, A. Schmidtke, & R. Wetz, pp. 121–29. Berlin: Springer.

Weisæth, L. (1988). Panikklidelse. *Medicinsk Årbog*, pp. 9–14. Copenhagen: Munksgaard.

Welz, R. (1988). Life events, current social stressors, and risk of attempted suicide. In *Current issues of suicidology*, ed. H.-J. Möller, A. Schmidtke & R. Welz, pp. 301–10. Berlin: Springer.

Welz, R., Veivel, T. O. & Häfner, H. (1988). Social support and suicidal behaviour. In *Current issues of suicidology*, ed. H.-J. Möller, A. Schmidtke & R. Welz, pp. 322–7. Berlin: Springer.

Wolfersdorf, M., Vogel, R. & Hole, G. (1985). Suizid in vier psychiatrischen Landes-krankenhäusern Baden-Würtenbergs. In *Suizidgefahr*, ed. V. Faust & M. Wolfersdorf, pp. 187–206. Stuttgart: Hippokrates.

Wolk-Wassermann, D. (1986). *Attempted suicide – the patient's family, social network and therapy*. Stockholm: Akademisk avhandling, Karolinska Institutet.

Wolk-Wassermann, D. (1988). Suicidal patients' comprehension of significant others' attitudes towards them. In *Current issues of suicidology*, ed. H.-J. Möller, A. Schmidtke & R. Welz, pp. 381–89. Berlin: springer.

World Health Organization (WHO) (1977). *International classification of diseases*. 9th revised edn. ICD-9. Geneva: World Health Organization.

World Health Organization (WHO) (1986). *Working group on preventive practices in suicide and attempted suicides*. Summary report (ICP/PSF 017 6526V). Copenhagen: WHO Regional Office for Europe.

Ziporyn, T. (1983). Depression, violent suicide tied to low metabolite level. *J. Am. Med. Assoc.*, **250**, 3141–2.

Åsberg, M. (1983). Psychobiologisk forskning kring depression och självmord. *Läkartidn*, **80**, 2508–9.

Åsberg, M. & Nordstrøm, P. (1988). Biological correlates of suicidal behaviour. In *Current issues of suicidology*, ed. H.-J. Möller, A. Schmidtke & R. Welz, pp. 221–41. Berlin: Springer.

Åsberg, M., Mårtensson, D. & Wägner, A. (1984). *Psychobiological aspects of suicidal behaviour*. Symposium on Psychopathology in the Perspective of Person-Environment Interaction, Stockholm 1984.

Index

self-destruction (*cont.*)
  organ removal, 7
  parts of body, 7
self-neglect
  'chronically suicidal', 5–6
  of physical disorder treatment, 7–8
Seneca, suicide, 15
senile brain disorders and suicide, 110
senior physicians, availability, 208
seppuku, 11
serotonin turnover, mental illness and
    suicide, 131, 132
sex
  and danger of suicide, 142
  incidence
    attempted suicide, Nordic countries,
      61–4
    suicide rate, Norway (1970–87), 50–5
  ratio for suicide, 75–6
  specification and suicide, 71
  suicide incidence, Greenland, 58–9, 60
  suicide rate
    Scandinavia, 52–3
    various groups, 55–8
shame, and suicide risk, 146
Shintoism and suicide, 11–12
shooting as method, 92, 94
sick persons, expected suicide, 9
single parentage and suicide, 76
  importance, 126–7
slashing arm as method, 99
sleeplessness and suicide risk, 146
social conditions and suicide rate, 30
social deprivation and suicide, 81
social factors triggering suicide, 80–90
social groups and suicide, 155
social or institutionalised suicide, 9
social integration, 70–1, 125
social isolation, 22
social services
  contact with suicidal patient, 204
  treatment, 156–9
socio-cultural factors, and suicide risk,
    151–2
sociological and demographic theories on
    lower suicide rate in Norway, 67–
    9
  comparison with other countries, 67–9
somatic hospitals
  management of suicidal patient, 205–6
  see also general hospital
SOS service of the church, 217
South America, statistics, 26
Spain, statistics, 26
starvation, suicide by, 10
statistics, 1–2, 25–44
  Canada, 27–30
  Catholic countries, 25–6

European countries, 26–7
Hungary, 26–7
Protestant countries, 25–6
suicide, 224
trends, 30–44
USA, 27–30
see also rate
status integration and suicide rate, 89–90
Stengel Prize, 223
Stoic School, attitude to suicide, 14–15
students, suicide rate, 82–3
substances used for poisoning, 95–9
sudden unexpected death and suicide
    registration, 70
suicidal patients, is there a need for
    separate institutions, 216–17
suicide
  altruistic, 20
  anomic, 20
  attempted, *see* attempted suicide:
    parasuicide
  and attempted suicide, as entirely
    different conditions, 200–1
  chronically suicidal, definition, 5–6
  definitions, 2, 4–5
  double, definition, 6
  egoistic, 20
  extended (complex), 6
  focal (local), 7
  in hospital wards, 164, 208–9
  messages, definition, 4
  with multifactorial causes, 8
  occurrence in ward, 164, 208–9
  once-off phenomenon, 6
  organic, 7–8
  prevention centres, 174–5
    the American approach, 219–20
  process, 4–5, 135–41
    ambivalence stage, 138
    decisive stage, 139
    deliberation stage, 138
    development from thoughts to act,
      135–7
    much deliberation or spontaneity,
      136–7, 138
    overall picture, 140–2
    presuicidal syndrome, 137–9
    probability of someone intervening,
      141–2
    probability of survival, 141–2
    start at any age, 137
    strain on family, 137
    as symbolic act, 136
  rate, 5
  recognised, in Buddhism, 11
    China, 11
    in Hinduism, 10
    Japanese culture, 11–12

nu